Toward Integrated DoD Biosurveillance

Assessment and Opportunities

Melinda Moore, Gail Fisher, Clare Stevens

Prepared for the United States Army
Approved for public release; distribution unlimited

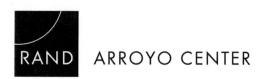

RAND ARROYO CENTER

The research described in this report was sponsored by the United States Army under Contract No. W74V8H-06-C-0001.

Library of Congress Cataloging-in-Publication Data is available for this publication.

ISBN 978-0-8330-8151-3

The RAND Corporation is a nonprofit institution that helps improve policy and decisionmaking through research and analysis. RAND's publications do not necessarily reflect the opinions of its research clients and sponsors.

Support RAND—make a tax-deductible charitable contribution at www.rand.org/giving/contribute.html

RAND® is a registered trademark.

RAND OFFICES
SANTA MONICA, CA • WASHINGTON, DC
PITTSBURGH, PA • NEW ORLEANS, LA • JACKSON, MS • BOSTON, MA
DOHA, QA • CAMBRIDGE, UK • BRUSSELS, BE
www.rand.org

Preface

Biosurveillance is a cornerstone of public health. In July 2012, the White House issued the National Strategy for Biosurveillance, which defines the term and sets out key functions and guiding principles. The Department of Defense (DoD) carries out biosurveillance to monitor the health of military and affiliated populations and supports biosurveillance in other countries through a range of programs across the department. The Deputy Secretary of Defense issued interim guidance in June 2013 for implementation of the new National Strategy. This begins to set formal policy for DoD's biosurveillance enterprise.

The Office of Management and Budget (OMB) recognized the importance of effective DoD biosurveillance not only for the department itself but also within the context of the National Strategy. With this in mind, OMB tasked DoD to carry out a comprehensive examination of its biosurveillance enterprise to determine priority missions and desired outcomes, the extent to which DoD biosurveillance programs contribute to these missions, and whether the current funding system is appropriate and how it can be improved to ensure stable funding. DoD leaders designated the Armed Forces Health Surveillance Center (AFHSC) to lead this assessment effort. AFHSC sought objective external analytic support from the RAND Arroyo Center, a component of the RAND Corporation, to respond to the tasks specified by OMB.

This report addresses the three OMB tasks. As such, it should be of interest to DoD policy makers and DoD components directly and indirectly involved in DoD's biosurveillance programming. It is also relevant to other federal policy makers across the range of departments and agencies that have responsibilities for domestic and global disease detection and response, and associated capacity building and intelligence—in particular the U.S. Departments of Health and Human Services, Homeland Security, and State, as well as the federal Intelligence Community. The report should also be of interest to the U.S. Congress and others who seek to improve the efficiency and effectiveness of biosurveillance across the federal government.

This research was sponsored by AFHSC within DoD and conducted by the RAND Arroyo Center. The Arroyo Center is a federally funded research and development center sponsored by the Department of the Army.

For more information on the Arroyo Center, see http://www.rand.org/ard.html or contact the Director, Mr. Timothy Bonds (contact information is provided on the web page). For more information specifically on the Army Health Program, please contact the Director, Dr. Margaret Harrell, or the Assistant Director, Dr. Sarah Meadows (contact information also on the web page).

Comments or questions on this report should be addressed to the project leader, Dr. Melinda Moore, who can be reached by email at Melinda_Moore@rand.org or by phone at 703-413-1100, x5234.

Table of Contents

Figures

Tables

Summary

The purpose of this study is to examine the missions and performance of the Department of Defense (DoD) biosurveillance enterprise. Specifically, the Office of Management and Budget (OMB) asked DoD to undertake a comprehensive review of its biosurveillance activities to accomplish the following tasks:

- Task 1: Identify a prioritized list of the program's missions and desired outcomes, and develop performance measures and targets to track progress toward achieving those outcomes.
- Task 2: Evaluate how the current array of DoD biosurveillance program assets contributes to achieving these prioritized missions.
- Task 3: Assess whether the current funding system is appropriate and how it can be improved to assure stable funding.

Public health surveillance is a cornerstone of public health—an "essential function of a public health system" (Nsubuga, 2006)—just as national security surveillance and analysis are a cornerstone of national security. Health security is at the nexus where public health and national security meet. Public health surveillance typically reflects all hazards occurring in human populations, whether naturally occurring, accidental, or intentional.

Biosurveillance is more expansive in scope than public health surveillance because it applies to "all-hazards threats ... affecting human, animal or plant health." Different agencies and earlier national policy documents use different definitions of biosurveillance. The one used in this study is from the National Strategy for Biosurveillance, dated July 2012. This definition of biosurveillance places an emphasis on the use of information for early detection and warning of events that are the "result of a bioterror attack or other weapons of mass destruction threat, an emerging infectious disease, pandemic, environmental disaster, or a food-borne illness." Moreover, the Strategy also highlights a need to protect "domestic interests, and because health threats transcend national borders, the United States also plays a vital role within an international network of biosurveillance centers across the globe."

The interim guidance for implementation of the National Strategy for Biosurveillance, issued by the Deputy Secretary of Defense on June 13, 2013, was the first DoD policy guidance referring explicitly to "biosurveillance." It indicates that DoD adopts the Strategy's definition of the term, calls for development of a DoD Directive (DoDD) on biosurveillance within 12 months, and specifies early tasks and a governance mechanism, pending the Directive. In the present report, DoD's "biosurveillance enterprise" refers to the programs, policies, and funding related to biosurveillance activities—drawing from the definition of the term and the functions and guiding principles of the National Strategy for Biosurveillance—and the DoD organizations responsible for such activities.

DoD has been conducting biosurveillance activities for several years through entities under three main stakeholders within the Office of the Secretary of Defense (OSD)—the Under Secretaries of Defense for Protection and Readiness; Acquisition, Technology and Logistics; and Intelligence—and the Services. The enterprise encompasses a wide range of relevant activities, from traditional health surveillance to medical intelligence, host nation biosurveillance capacity building, and defense against biological weapons.

The focus of the DoD biosurveillance enterprise is on human health (and less on animal or plant disease), which is aligned with the core defense missions of providing the forces needed to deter war and protect the homeland (DoD, 2012b). Therefore, it is not surprising that a central and traditional element of the biosurveillance enterprise is the set of human health surveillance activities related to Service members and affiliated populations, as well as occupational and environmental health surveillance, carried out by the Services, the Armed Forces Health Surveillance Center (AFHSC), and DoD laboratories in the continental United States (CONUS) and outside the continental United States (OCONUS).

DoD's Intelligence Community provides additional value to the biosurveillance enterprise. It uses intelligence tradecraft to provide "early warning" to identify and forecast emerging and potentially destabilizing threats. Medical intelligence activities are carried out under the Defense Intelligence Agency's (DIA's) National Center for Medical Intelligence (NCMI).

Work under the Assistant Secretary of Defense for Nuclear, Chemical, and Biological Defense Programs (ASD [NCB]), aimed at countering biological weapons, focuses on helping countries build their physical and professional biosurveillance capacity and capabilities. This includes technological acquisitions and cooperative biological research, which contribute to both global health security and a strategic engagement strategy. Program activities generally involve assisting prioritized countries with building laboratories, training epidemiologists, and using surveillance strategies and tools appropriately for effective health surveillance.

The DoD biosurveillance enterprise undertakes a variety of biosurveillance activities in the United States and internationally, for a range of customers and purposes. It monitors health in military populations and military families in CONUS and deployed populations, including civilians and contractors. It also supports collaborative surveillance with foreign governments in countries and regions of interest, for those countries' own situational awareness and reporting. As noted earlier, the entire enterprise looks for hazards that are natural and/or manmade to both protect the forces and detect potential biological weapons threats, as well as to enhance global health security more broadly. DoD, the U.S. government, and international policy makers and responders are the consumers of information produced by the DoD biosurveillance enterprise.

In order to respond to the tasks from OMB, the study team examined DoD's biosurveillance systems and assets, the enabling functions that support them (policy and doctrine, governance, organizational structures, personnel and training, materiel, logistics, and facilities), and the funding systems currently associated with the biosurveillance enterprise. They organized these using a logic model that flows from inputs (enabling functions and funding) to processes (biosurveillance systems and assets), outputs (reports and alerts), outcomes (desired outcomes from biosurveillance), and impacts (strategic missions served). The logic model elements track well with the three OMB tasks, as shown in Figure S.1.

Figure S.1. Logic Model for DoD Biosurveillance

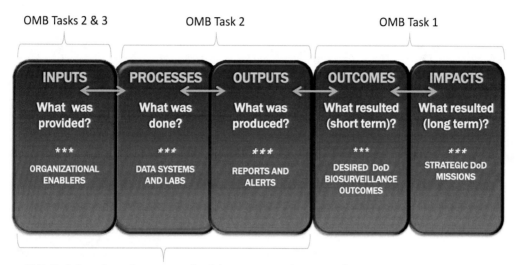

OMB Task 2 analyses focus on each of these separately, especially as they relate to desired outcomes and strategic DoD missions.

OMB Task 1: Identify a prioritized list of the program's missions and desired outcomes, and develop performance measures and targets to track progress toward achieving those outcomes.

The DoD biosurveillance enterprise is not comprised of a single program; hence, the study team examined the DoD strategic missions to which biosurveillance contributes and prioritized those missions. Based on review of U.S. statute and international law, national policy, and DoD doctrine/policy, the team determined that the highest-priority strategic DoD mission relevant to biosurveillance is force health protection, followed by biological weapons defense (which itself also supports force health protection), and global health security. The first two are Congressionally mandated, and the third is mandated by national (Executive Branch) policy and one binding international treaty. DoD biosurveillance supports all three of these missions (Figure S.2).

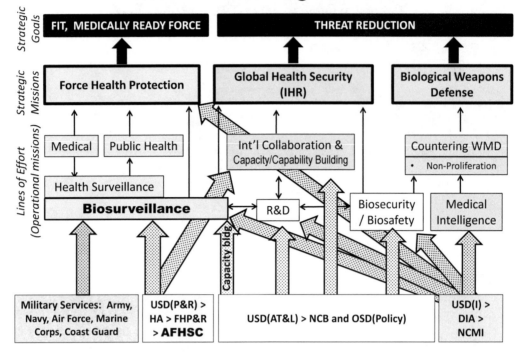

On June 27, 2013, the White House issued fiscal year 2015 budget guidance that specifies priorities related to the National Strategy for Countering Biological Threats and the associated Global Health Security second-term agenda. Specifically, it asks federal agencies, including DoD, to align their relevant fiscal year 2015 budget requests with the eight priority objectives under larger aims to (a) prevent avoidable epidemics, (b) detect threats early, and (c) respond rapidly and effectively to biological threats of international concern. This issuance underscores the importance that the White House attaches to a U.S. global health security mission.

The National Strategy for Biosurveillance, issued in July 2012, suggests desired outcomes for biosurveillance. These are relevant to DoD biosurveillance as well:

- Early warning of threats and early detection of events
- Situational awareness
- Decision making at all levels, including acute response, policy, and research and development
- Forecast of impacts.

DoD biosurveillance supports the three strategic-level missions and four desired outcomes:

- NCMI in particular provides indicators and early warning and forecasting of impact
- AFHSC's Global Emerging Infections Surveillance and Response System (GEIS), NCMI, and the Cooperative Biological Engagement Program (CBEP) all contribute to

situational awareness globally; the Services and AFHSC's biosurveillance support situational awareness among military Service members
- All components of the DoD biosurveillance enterprise enable decision making by DoD, the U.S. government, and host nation officials

Biosurveillance programs can be prioritized based on the relative priority of these three strategic-level missions, with programs supporting force health protection accorded the highest priority.

Performance measures can monitor relevant actions, outputs, and outcomes. Development of performance measures and targets typically requires intensive efforts over months or years, but the study team identified a number of potentially relevant measures to be considered.

OMB Task 2: Evaluate how the current array of DoD biosurveillance program assets contributes to achieving these prioritized missions.

Assessment of the performance of DoD biosurveillance processes (systems and laboratories) indicates the following:

- DoD biosurveillance population and data coverage for military Service members are comprehensive; biosurveillance in Service members supports DoD's force health protection mission.
- DoD biosurveillance population and data coverage internationally cover syndromes and pathogens of relevance to partner countries and to DoD; international biosurveillance supports both the force health protection and global health security missions of DoD and also the broader U.S. government and global health security communities.
- The quality of DoD biosurveillance is higher than typical public health surveillance because of the availability of denominator data, standardized case definitions, and the high quality and high degree of testing performed by DoD laboratories.
- Very little data analysis by AFHSC is oriented to near-real-time situational awareness. More frequent (e.g., more daily) analyses and some additional data linkages could further enhance the value of DoD biosurveillance used for situational awareness purposes.

AFHSC produces more than 1,000 distinct recurrent reports each year, plus ad hoc reports and journal publications (65 articles published in AFHSC's *Medical Surveillance Monthly Report* and 60 additional papers published in peer-reviewed journals during fiscal year 2012). AFHSC produces no routine near-real-time reports for situational awareness purposes, although the final operating capability of its Division of Integrated Biosurveillance (DIB) envisages daily analysis and reporting, if resources become available. In contrast, NCMI presently conducts daily scans of 70–80 diseases of military interest across 165 countries, and produces reports from these.

Analysis of inputs (enabling functions) suggests that personnel shortages are likely the most significant hindrance to formalization and expansion of the biosurveillance enterprise capabilities and capacities. The AFHSC's chain of command (the Assistant Secretary of Defense [Health Affairs] or ASD[HA]) signed a Memorandum of Understanding (MOU) with the ASD(NCB) in 2012. The MOU recognizes AFHSC as the center for the emerging biosurveillance capability. In

2012, AFHSC established the DIB to oversee integration of biosurveillance efforts across DoD. The limiting enabler for the AFHSC—and therefore for the entire enterprise—is manpower within the DIB, which currently has only seven staff members. AFHSC currently has a total of 78 staff, which is sufficient to sustain current operations but not the added responsibilities associated with the MOU. Most of those new responsibilities fall under the DIB. Furthermore, the staff expertise required for the DIB is considerable: qualifications include significant DoD experience as well as a high level of epidemiological expertise. AFHSC's current facilities can accommodate only 96 work spaces, not sufficient for the number of staff reflected in either past years of requests (110) or the February 2012 workload survey (134). Finally, AFHSC does not have its own classified terminals or classified computing facilities, which would enable it to better support integration across the DoD biosurveillance enterprise.

OMB Task 3: Assess whether the current funding system is appropriate and how it can be improved to assure stable funding.

DoD has a considerable investment in the biosurveillance enterprise. However, because there is no authority for a biosurveillance enterprise at the time of this report, there is no oversight mechanism for allocation of funds across the entire enterprise in a way to meet overarching goals and emerging needs. The funding systems that support each of the contributing organizations function well within those particular domains; however, there is no overall funding system.

Regarding stability, the Office of the ASD(NCB) has indicated that it expects relatively stable funding going forward in spite of the vulnerabilities and variations caused by the current cutbacks. NCMI is expecting significant cuts but does not anticipate a major compromise to its biosurveillance-related mission. AFHSC funding has been relatively stable in recent years, but, as noted above, current levels are insufficient for the additional responsibilities reflected in the MOU, according to AFHSC leaders. Moreover, formalization of the DoD biosurveillance enterprise—as reflected in the interim guidance issued by the Deputy Secretary of Defense on June 13, 2013, and the DoDD to follow in 12 months—could result in additional mission responsibilities for AFHSC. Because most of the new responsibilities under the MOU fall to AFHSC and the DIB, the near-term adequacy of AFHSC funding to fulfill both current and new responsibilities is more vulnerable than for the other key components of the DoD biosurveillance enterprise.

While there may still be funding shortages across the DoD biosurveillance enterprise, it is not inconceivable that agencies could share resources to advance common objectives. The entire enterprise would likely benefit from an oversight organization—for example, comprised of those charged to coordinate the tasks specified in the June 2013 interim guidance—to determine the feasibility and appropriateness of resource sharing, examine redundancies, and routinely review and synchronize the efforts of the stakeholders within the resource realities of the department.

In conclusion, well-integrated DoD biosurveillance can provide effective, efficient, and important support to all three relevant DoD strategic missions. These missions are, in turn, consistent with higher-level national health, security, and health security policy. Information from biosurveillance, as from any public health surveillance, "improves the efficiency and effectiveness of health services by targeting interventions and documenting their effect on the population" (Nsubuga, 2006). Absent formal cost-effectiveness analysis of the DoD biosurveillance enterprise, it is reasonable to conclude that modest marginal investments toward a more integrated and efficient DoD biosurveillance enterprise will yield positive returns to both DoD and the larger national and international community in health, economic, and global health security terms. AFHSC is well-positioned to serve as an effective hub for integrated DoD biosurveillance, but it appears to need additional staff and enhanced facilities to more robustly fulfill its current and potential future responsibilities. This is already important as AFHSC assumes additional responsibilities under the MOU between ASD(HA) and ASD(NCB) and will become increasingly important as biosurveillance is formally defined in DoD doctrine/policy and AFHSC's activities are aligned with the National Strategy for Biosurveillance, the priorities specified in the June 2013 budget guidance for fiscal year 2015, and the associated Global Health Security second-term agenda.

Acknowledgments

Many people gave generously of their time and expertise in support of this project. Our great appreciation goes to CAPT Kevin Russell, Director of the Armed Forces Health Surveillance Center (AFHSC), and AFHSC staff members who met with us on several occasions to provide information and feedback that were important to our efforts. In this regard, we thank Dr. Kelly Vest, Deputy Chief of Staff-Operations, who served as our principal contact in AFHSC; Dr. Rohit Chitale, Director of the Division of Integrated Biosurveillance (DIB); LCDR Jean-Paul Chretien, Assistant Director of the DIB; and Mr. Robert Welch, Executive Officer/Chief of Staff.

We also wish to thank staff members from other DoD offices for their time and insights, specifically Col Steven Niehoff from the Office of the Deputy Assistant Secretary of Defense for Force Health Protection and Readiness; Dr. Ben Petro and Dr. Julia Dooher from the Office of the Assistant Secretary of Defense for Chemical and Biological Defense Programs; Mr. Lance Brooks, Dr. Carl Newman, Dr. Jeffrey Fields, and Mr. Mike Keifer from the Cooperative Biological Engagement Program; and staff with whom we met from the National Center for Medical Intelligence.

We thank the RAND researchers who reviewed this report as part of RAND's Quality Assurance process and provided comprehensive and thoughtful feedback: the two formal reviewers, Dr. Jeanne Ringel and Ms. Kathryn Connor, and also Dr. Rick Eden, RAND Arroyo Center's Research Quality Assurance Manager, as well as LTC Michael Franco, an Army Medical Command officer and Army Fellow with RAND from 2012–2013. Finally, we are indebted to our RAND colleagues Dr. Margaret Harrell and Dr. Sarah Meadows, Director and Associate Director (respectively) of the Arroyo Health Program, for their supportive and helpful oversight.

Abbreviations

AFEB	Armed Forces Epidemiology Board
AFHSC	Armed Forces Health Surveillance Center
AFRIMS	Armed Forces Research Institute of Medical Sciences
AFRRI	Armed Forces Radiobiology Research Institute
AHLTA	Armed Forces Health Longitudinal Technology Application
ASD(HA)	Assistant Secretary of Defense (Health Affairs)
ASD(NCB)	Assistant Secretary of Defense (Nuclear, Chemical and Biological Defense Programs)
ASPR	Assistant Secretary for Preparedness and Response (within HHS)
AT&L	Acquisition, Technology and Logistics
CBEP	Cooperative Biological Engagement Program
CCMD	Combatant Command
CDC	Centers for Disease Control and Prevention
CDD	Centers for Disease Detection
CNO	Chief of Naval Operations
CONOPS	concept of operations
CONUS	continental United States
CTR	Cooperative Threat Reduction
DASD(FHP&R)	Deputy Assistant Secretary of Defense for Force Health Protection and Readiness
DHA	Defense Health Agency
DHS	Department of Homeland Security
DHSS	Defense Health Services Systems
DIA	Defense Intelligence Agency
DIB	Division of Integrated Biosurveillance
DMSS	Defense Medical Surveillance System
DMTS	Division of Data Management and Technical Support

DoD	Department of Defense
DoDD	Department of Defense Directive
DoDI	Department of Defense Instruction
DoDSR	Department of Defense Serum Repository
DOEHRS	Defense Occupational and Environmental Health Readiness System
DOTMLPF	doctrine, organization, training, materiel, leadership and education, personnel, and facilities
DRSi	Disease Reporting System internet
DTRA	Defense Threat Reduction Agency
EPMU	Environmental Preventive Medicine Unit (U.S. Navy)
ESSENCE	Electronic Surveillance System for the Early Notification of Community-based Epidemics
FDA	Food and Drug Administration
FHP	force health protection
GEIS	Global Emerging Infections Surveillance and Response System
HHS	Department of Health and Human Services
HSPD	Homeland Security Presidential Directive
IHR	International Health Regulations
JBAIDS	Joint Biological Agent Identification and Diagnostic System
JMEWS	Joint Medical Workstation
JPEO	joint program executive office
JRO	Joint Requirements Office
JSTO	Joint Science and Technology Office
JUPITR	Joint USFK Portal and Integrated Threat Recognition
JWICS	Joint Worldwide Intelligence Computing System
MEDCOM	U.S. Army Medical Command
MEPS	Military Entrance Processing Station
MHS	Military Health System
MOA	Memorandum of Agreement
MoD	Ministry of Defense

MoH	Ministry of Health
MOU	Memorandum of Understanding
MRMC	Medical Research and Materiel Command (U.S. Army)
MSMR	*Medical Surveillance Monthly Report*
MTF	military treatment facility
NAMRU	Navy Medical Research Unit
NATO	North Atlantic Treaty Organization
NBC	nuclear, biological, and chemical
NCMI	National Center for Medical Intelligence
NGDS	Next Generation Diagnostics System
NHRC	Naval Health Research Center
NMCPHC	Navy and Marine Corps Public Health Center
NMRC	Navy Medical Research Center
NSTC	National Science and Technology Council
OCONUS	outside the continental United States
ODNI	Office of the Director of National Intelligence
OMB	Office of Management and Budget
OSD	Office of the Secretary of Defense
OSD(P&R)	Office of the Under Secretary of Secretary of Defense (Personnel and Readiness)
PDD	Presidential Decision Directive
PHI	Public Health Infrastructure
POM	Program Objective Memorandum
PPD	Presidential Policy Directive
R&D	research and development
RDT&E	research, development, test, and evaluation
RME	reportable medical event
SIPRnet	Secure Internet Protocol Router Network
TMA	Tricare Management Activity
USAFRICOM	U.S. Africa Command

USAFSAM	U.S. Air Force School of Aerospace Medicine
USAMRICD	U.S. Army Medical Research Institute of Chemical Disease
USAMRIID	U.S. Army Medical Research Institute for Infectious Diseases
USAMRU	U.S. Army Medical Research Unit
USAPHC	U.S. Army Public Health Command
USCENTCOM	U.S. Central Command
USCG	U.S. Coast Guard
USD(AT&L)	Under Secretary of Defense (Acquisition, Technology, and Logistics)
USD(I)	Under Secretary of Defense (Intelligence)
USD(P&R)	Under Secretary of Defense (Personnel and Readiness)
USEUCOM	U.S. European Command
USNORTHCOM	U.S. Northern Command
USPACOM	U.S. Pacific Command
USSOUTHCOM	U.S. Southern Command
USTRANSCOM	U.S. Transportation Command
USUHS	Uniformed Services University of the Health Sciences
VA	Department of Veterans Affairs
WHO	World Health Organization
WMD	weapons of mass destruction
WRAIR	Walter Reed Army Institute of Research

1. Introduction

Public Health Surveillance Is a Cornerstone of Public Health, National Security, and Health Security

HEALTH · HEALTH SECURITY · SECURITY

Public health surveillance

National security surveillance & analysis

- **Health security:** Health security is a state in which the Nation and its people are prepared for, protected from, and resilient in the face of health threats or incidents with potentially negative health consequences *(NHSS, 2009)*
- **Public health surveillance:** Systematic, ongoing collection, analysis, interpretation and dissemination of data for public health action *(Thacker, 2000)*

Source: Figure adapted from CDC "Public Health Preparedness Capabilities", 2010 (page 3)

Public health surveillance is a cornerstone of public health, just as national security surveillance and analysis is a cornerstone of national security.

Health security is at the nexus where public health and national security meet. The 2009 National Health Security Strategy defines *health security* as

> a state in which the Nation and its people are prepared for, protected from, and resilient in the face of health threats or incidents with potentially negative health consequences. (HHS, 2009)

One of the most widely cited definitions of *public health surveillance* is

> The *systematic collection, analysis, interpretation*, and dissemination of data regarding a health-related event *for use in public health action* to reduce morbidity and mortality and to improve health. (Thacker, 2000; emphasis added)

Another definition from the Institute of Medicine is similar but adds an important dimension:

> *ongoing systematic collection, analysis*, and *interpretation* of health data, essential to the *planning, implementation, and evaluation of public health practice*, closely integrated to the dissemination of these data to those who need to know and *linked to prevention and control*. (Institute of Medicine, 2002; emphasis added)

The added emphases highlight some of the key features of public health surveillance: its systematic and ongoing nature, the inclusion of data interpretation as well as data analysis, and

1

the intention that surveillance directly inform public health action. "Health data" and "health-related events" refer to health monitoring for routine public health prevention and management purposes, as explicitly indicated in the second definition, as well as to detecting anomalous trends or acute incidents such as disease outbreaks that require specific response. Although not explicit in the definitions, the threats under public health surveillance typically reflect all hazards—they can be naturally occurring as well as accidental or intentional. Also not explicit in the definitions is that public health surveillance traditionally has referred principally to health monitoring in human populations (and not in animals or plants).

"Biosurveillance" is more expansive than, and encompasses, "public health surveillance." Different agencies and earlier national policy documents use different definitions of biosurveillance (see Table 1.1). The definition used in this study is from the National Strategy for Biosurveillance, dated July 2012. This definition places an emphasis on the use of information for early detection and warning of events which are the

> result of a bioterror attack or other weapons of mass destruction threat, an emerging infectious disease, pandemic, environmental disaster, or a food-borne illness. (p. 1)

Moreover, the Strategy also highlights a need to protect

> domestic interests, and because health threats transcend national borders, the United States also plays a vital role within an international network of biosurveillance centers across the globe. (p. 1)

Finally, the definition specifies the scope as

> all-hazards threats ... affecting human, animal or plant health.

Thus, this definition is more expansive by explicitly including all hazards, and not only human, but also animal and plant health. This broader scope is important and will be used later in this report to frame how the study team examined the DoD biosurveillance enterprise.

Table 1.1. Different Definitions of Biosurveillance

Source	Definition
National Strategy for Biosurveillance (2012)	"the process of gathering, integrating, interpreting, and communicating essential information related to all-hazards threats or disease activity affecting human, animal, or plant health to achieve early detection and warning, contribute to overall situational awareness of the health aspects of an incident, and to enable better decision making at all levels."
Homeland Security Presidential Directive (HSPD)-21 Public Health and Medical Preparedness (2007)	"the process of active data-gathering with appropriate analysis and interpretation of biosphere data that might relate to disease activity and threats to human or animal health—whether infectious, toxic, metabolic, or otherwise, and regardless of intentional or natural origin—in order to achieve early warning of health threats, early detection of health events, and overall situational awareness of disease activity"
Centers for Disease Control and Prevention (CDC) National Biosurveillance Strategy for Human Health (2011)	"the science and practice of managing health-related data and information for early warning of threats and hazards, early detection of events, and rapid characterization of the event so that effective actions can be taken to mitigate adverse health effects. Biosurveillance represents a new health information paradigm for public health that seeks to integrate and efficiently manage health-related data and information across a range of information systems with the primary goal of timely and accurate population health situation awareness."

**The National Strategy for Biosurveillance (2012)
Establishes Core Functions and Guiding Principles**

NATIONAL STRATEGY
FOR BIOSURVEILLANCE

Four core functions

- Scan and discern the environment
- Identify and integrate essential information
- Alert and inform decision makers
- Forecast and advise impacts

Four guiding principles

- Leverage existing capabilities
- Embrace an all-of-Nation approach
- Add value for all participants
- Maintain a global perspective

The 2012 National Strategy for Biosurveillance establishes not only a national definition for biosurveillance but also four core functions and four guiding principles. These are relevant to consideration of the missions, outcomes, and programs associated with the DoD biosurveillance enterprise:

- Four core functions

    - Scan and discern the environment: Key to this function is the scope of information that includes not only human health, but also animal, plant, and environmental health, all of which may contribute to core biosurveillance functions. Key characteristics include constant scanning of the environment and rapid evaluation to detect threats and assess their severity.

    - Identify and integrate essential information: This function focuses on the identification, sharing, and integration of information for detection and assessment purposes. Key to this function is the idea that information should be integrated from disparate information sources, such as intelligence data, law enforcement sources, and plant, animal, and environmental sources. It also implicitly encompasses the notion of the transformation of "data" into actionable "information."

    - Alert and inform decision makers: This function directs that key decision makers be informed of potential threats in a timely fashion, even if action might not be warranted.

    - Forecast and advise impacts: Decisions often require forecasting of future impacts. This function focuses on the ability to identify most likely/probable impacts and outcomes of any incident as well as the most dangerous and worst case scenarios.

- Four guiding principles

    - Leverage existing capabilities: Harness and use existing systems; avoid redundancies.

- Embrace an all-of-Nation approach: Involve all relevant actors, including relevant federal agencies.
- Add value for all participants: Minimize burden, enable efficiencies, and make surveillance information valuable at the community level.
- Maintain a global perspective: This recognizes that biological agents and events are not neatly and inherently contained within national borders, and that therefore a global perspective is essential to a U.S. national strategy for biosurveillance

Further, DoD's biosurveillance enterprise is nested within the context of recent national strategies (Figure 1.1) as well as the World Health Organization's (WHO's) International Health Regulations (IHR 2005), which call for countries to develop, maintain, and operationalize core capacities to detect, report, and respond to public health emergencies of international concern (WHO, 2008).

Figure 1.1. DoD Biosurveillance in a Larger National and International Context

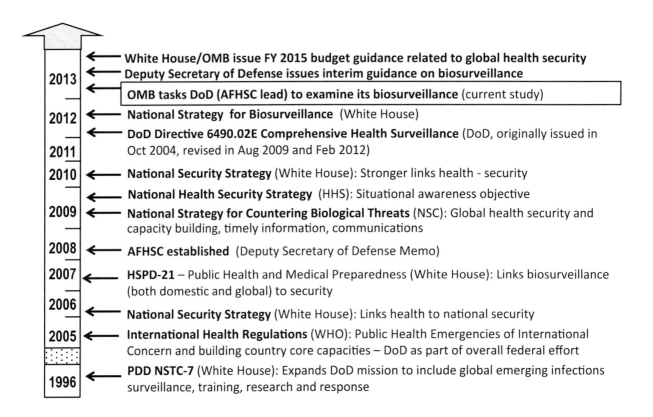

The 1996 Presidential Decision Directive (PDD) National Science and Technology Council (NSTC)-7 stemmed from the U.S. government's global strategy to address emerging infectious diseases, which called for DoD to expand its mission to include surveillance, training, research, and response in this area. The Global Emerging Infections Surveillance and Response System (GEIS) was created in response to this directive.

The 2006 National Security Strategy was the first such strategy to link health—the threat of pandemic disease—to national security (White House, 2006). The National Security Strategy of 2010 encompasses an even more robust range of health system and public health issues to national security (White House, 2010).

HSPD "Public Health and Medical Preparedness" (2007) linked domestic and global biosurveillance to security (HSPD 21, 2007).

The National Strategy for Countering Biological Threats drew explicit attention to promoting *global health security*: helping countries build their capacity to detect, identify, and report outbreaks; ensure timely situational awareness; and communicate effectively at all levels, as well as a number of objectives related to reduce the proliferation of biological threats (PDD 2, 2009).

The 2009 National Health Security Strategy includes cross-border and global cooperation as one of its ten objectives and situational awareness as another objective (HHS, 2009).

The 2012 National Strategy for Biosurveillance further focuses on biosurveillance in particular, drawing from these higher-order security-oriented national policy documents (White House, 2012).

The DoD biosurveillance enterprise functions within the context of these national strategies and the WHO IHR, as well as serving the military's own relevant strategic and operational missions under DoD-specific doctrine and policy.

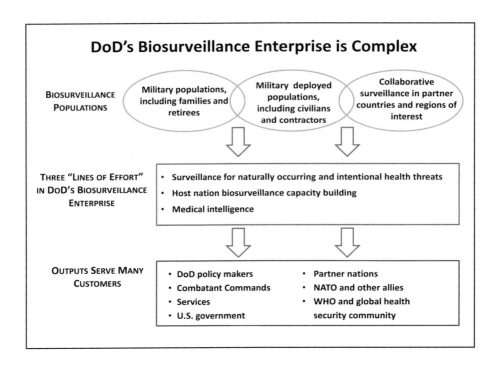

DoD has been conducting biosurveillance activities for several years. However, until the June 2013 interim guidance issued by the Deputy Secretary of Defense, which specified that the department adopt the definition in the National Strategy for Biosurveillance, DoD had no official definition of biosurveillance. Biosurveillance activities have not always been defined as such (see Chapter Two section on Missions for further discussion of biosurveillance and related definitions); this report refers to these activities as "lines of effort." These lines of effort are aligned to the core defense missions of providing the forces needed to deter war and protect the homeland (DoD, 2012b).

This report uses the term "DoD biosurveillance enterprise" to refer to all biosurveillance-related programs, policies, and funding, as well as the associated organizational components responsible for them. The enterprise samples different populations, uses different approaches, and has a wide range of customers and purposes. It samples military populations and military families in CONUS and deployed populations, including civilians and contractors OCONUS. It also supports the efforts of partner countries to carry out biosurveillance activities for their own situational awareness and reporting purposes. The entire enterprise looks for hazards that are natural and/or manmade. DoD, the U.S. government, and international policy makers and responders are the consumers of information produced by and through the DoD biosurveillance enterprise.

The purpose of this study is to examine the missions and performance of the DoD biosurveillance enterprise. Specifically, the Office of Management and Budget (OMB) requested that DoD undertake a comprehensive review of its biosurveillance activities to accomplish the following tasks:

- <u>Task 1</u>: Identify a prioritized list of the program's missions and desired outcomes, and develop performance measures and targets to track progress toward achieving those outcomes.
- <u>Task 2</u>: Evaluate how the current array of DoD biosurveillance program assets contributes to achieving these prioritized missions.
- <u>Task 3</u>: Assess whether the current funding system is appropriate and how it can be improved to assure stable funding.

DoD leadership tasked the Armed Forces Health Surveillance Center (AFHSC) to lead this assessment. AFHSC requested that the RAND Arroyo Center, a component of the RAND Corporation, examine the DoD biosurveillance enterprise in order to inform its response to the OMB.

DoD reached agreement with the OMB to submit its final report on August 16, 2013, rather than a preliminary report by June 30 (as originally requested) and a final report shortly thereafter.

> ## Methods: The Study Team Reviewed Documents and Met with Key DoD Biosurveillance Stakeholders
>
> - **Document review**
>   - AFHSC-related documents, provided by AFHSC (n ~30)
>   - One descriptive program document each provided by Cooperative Biological Engagement Program (CBEP), National Center for Medical Intelligence (NCMI)
>   - Independent identification by RAND of federal legislation, national policy/guidance documents, DoD doctrine/guidance, other U.S. government documents, international policy, published papers (n ~80)
> - **Meetings with key DoD stakeholders**
>   - AFHSC: Five on-site meetings, each with three to five AFHSC staff and one that also included a staff member from OSD(HA)/FHP&R
>   - CBEP: One discussion with four staff members
>   - OASD(CBD): One discussion with two staff members from the Office of the Assistant Secretary of Defense for Chemical and Biological Defense Programs
>   - NCMI: One discussion with three staff members
>   - Combatant Command: One discussion with two public health professionals in surgeon's office

To obtain the necessary information for its analyses, the study team reviewed documents and met with key DoD stakeholders. AFHSC provided approximately 30 internal reports, presentations, and other documents specifically related to AFHSC and DoD, and the Cooperative Biological Engagement Program (CBEP) and National Center for Medical Intelligence (NCMI) staff each provided one descriptive program document. The study team searched independently to identify authoritative sources from the U.S. Code, national policy documents, DoD doctrine/policy documents, DoD budget documents, other DoD documents, other relevant U.S. government and international documents, and relevant published journal papers—approximately 80 documents in all. Appendix A includes a full listing of documents reviewed by the study team.

In addition, the team met with AFHSC staff (during five onsite meetings and numerous follow-up communications) and once each (also onsite meetings) with DoD stakeholders from the office of the Assistant Secretary of Defense for Nuclear Chemical and Biological Defense Programs (ASD[NCB]), CBEP (under the Defense Threat Reduction Agency [DTRA]), NCMI (within the Defense Intelligence Agency [DIA]), and by phone with two public health professionals in one geographic Combatant Command (CCMD).

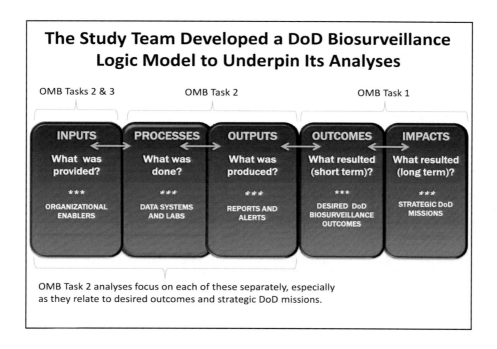

The study team developed a logic model to orient the organization of data collection. As described in a 2006 RAND report (Greenfield, 2006)

> The logic model inherently conceptualizes the relationship between program operations, strategies, and evidence, and, as such, can provide a framework to ensure that the evidence selected is consistent with the operations of a program as well as its strategic goals. We also note the importance of using the framework of the logic model to select evidence that supports causal linkages between the 'bins' in the logic model. (p. 20)

> The [logic] model can also be used to clearly identify program boundaries and delineate responsibilities, thereby clarifying the meaning of "impact" as it relates to the program. As such, a logic model can aid in program planning and evaluation…. For example, with regard to evaluation, a logic model itself can serve as evidence by providing a strong signal that a program understands its purpose and is "on track." (p. 6)

The study team developed a logic model specific to the conditions and requirements of the DoD biosurveillance enterprise and the OMB tasks. Specifically:

- Identification of desired biosurveillance outcomes and the impacts as reflected in DoD strategic missions address OMB Task 1; here, short-term refers to the timely and actionable outcomes that are typically directly related to specific surveillance information and outputs, whereas long-term refers to larger-order impacts that typically result from both surveillance information and the actions that follow.
- Identification and assessment of critical inputs (organizational enablers) and characterization and assessment of processes (data systems and laboratories) and biosurveillance outputs address OMB Task 2.
- Assessment of the appropriateness and stability of one particular input—such as funding—for the DoD biosurveillance enterprise addresses OMB Task 3.

The following chapters address each of the three OMB Tasks in turn (Chapters Two through Four), and the final chapter (Chapter Five) describes limitations and provides conclusions.

2. OMB Task 1—Missions and Outcomes

OMB Task 1: Identify a prioritized list of DoD biosurveillance programs, missions, desired outcomes, and associated performance measures and targets.

Findings:

- Based mostly on existing statute, force health protection is the top-priority mission related to biosurveillance, followed by biological weapons defense and global health security.
- The Global Health Security second-term agenda issued by the White House on June 27, 2013, underscores the priority attached to a U.S. global health security mission.
- The National Strategy for Biosurveillance suggests desired outcomes, and these are validated by other relevant sources.
- DoD biosurveillance supports the three strategic-level missions and four outcomes.
- Prioritization of strategic missions suggests that the highest-priority biosurveillance programs should be the 21 that address force health protection, followed by the one that addresses biological weapons defense (but not force health protection), and then the seven programs that address only global health security.

Methods

OMB Task 1: Identify a prioritized list of DoD biosurveillance programs, missions, desired outcomes, and associated performance measures and targets

- Review DoD documents and seek/examine authoritative sources to identify DoD missions relevant to biosurveillance
- Organize these missions from strategic to operational levels
- Develop and apply criteria to prioritize strategic missions
- Draw from list of DoD biosurveillance organizations and systems provided by AFHSC to identify DoD biosurveillance programs
- Link biosurveillance programs to strategic missions
- Draw from the National Strategy for Biosurveillance and other documents to identify desired biosurveillance outcomes
- Identify potential performance measures and targets

The first task from OMB was to identify a prioritized list of DoD biosurveillance programs, missions, desired outcomes, and associated performance measures and targets.

To identify DoD missions related to biosurveillance and/or the key DoD entities involved in the biosurveillance enterprise, the study team drew from reports and, where possible, authoritative sources. The project team then organized these in tiers from strategic down to operational levels. The team then developed and applied criteria to prioritize strategic-level missions. They selected the strategic-level missions for priority setting because all other relevant missions flow up to them.

To identify DoD biosurveillance programs, the team drew from a document provided by AFHSC that listed biosurveillance systems and their owner, purpose, and data frequency. They reconfigured the list into two separate tables: one for data systems and one for relevant biosurveillance assets, such as laboratories or capacity building programs. The team selectively deleted programs that are not directly related to biosurveillance data systems or assets, such as research and development (R&D) programs (which constitute a large part of the funding and activity in one of the major stakeholder entities but do not directly contribute to biosurveillance data). The team compiled the two lists and then classified each program (i.e., biosurveillance system or asset) according to one or more of the strategic-level mission each supports, based on documentation from the original AFHSC document. They also added one item to the list provided by AFHSC.

To identify desired outcomes from DoD biosurveillance, the study team examined the National Strategy for Biosurveillance and sought validation from other relevant sources. To identify potential performance measures, they reviewed internal DoD documents provided by AFHSC as well as national policy documents and published papers.

Missions

DoD Has Defined Different Types of Surveillance

- **Biosurveillance**
  - DoD adopted the definition from National Strategy for Biosurveillance (DepSecDef, 6/13/13): the process of gathering, *integrating,* interpreting, and communicating essential information related to *all-hazards* threats or disease activity affecting *human, animal, or plant health* to achieve early detection and warning, *contribute to overall situational awareness* of the health aspects of an incident, and to *enable better decisionmaking* at all levels

- **Health surveillance** (DoDD 6490.02E, 2012; JP 1-02):
  - The *regular or repeated* collection, analysis, and interpretation of health-related data and the dissemination of *information* to monitor the *health of a population* and to identify potential risks to health, thereby enabling timely interventions to prevent, treat, or control disease and injury. It includes *occupational and environmental health surveillance and medical surveillance*

- **Comprehensive health surveillance** (DoDD 6490.02E, 2012)
  - Health surveillance conducted *throughout Service members' military careers* and DoD civilian employees' employment, across all duty locations, and encompassing risk, intervention, and outcome data. Such surveillance is essential to the evaluation, planning, and implementation of public health practice and prevention and must be closely integrated with the *timely dissemination of information* to those who can *act upon it*

- **Medical surveillance** (DoDD 6490.02E, JP 1-02)
  - The ongoing, systematic collection, analysis, and interpretation of data derived from instances of *medical care or medical evaluation*, and *the reporting* of *population-based information* for *characterizing and countering threats* to a population's health, well-being, and performance

- **Medical intelligence** (DoDI 6420.01, 2009)
  - The product of collection, evaluation, and *all-source analysis* of *worldwide health threats and issues*, including foreign medical capabilities, infectious disease, environmental health risks, developments in biotechnology and biomedical subjects of national and military importance, and *support to force protection*

The Deputy Secretary of Defense's June 2013 interim guidance for implementing the National Strategy for Biosurveillance adopts the definition of biosurveillance from the Strategy. DoD has defined a number of other types of surveillance that are relevant to biosurveillance. The key and/or distinguishing features of each are highlighted below:

Biosurveillance (National Strategy for Biosurveillance, 2012)

> the process of gathering, *integrating,* interpreting, and communicating essential information related to all-hazards threats or disease activity affecting *human, animal, or plant health* to achieve *early detection and warning*, *contribute to overall situational awareness* of the health aspects of an incident, and to *enable better decision making* at all levels

Health surveillance (DoDD 6490.02E, 2012; Joint Publication 1-02, 2013)

> The *regular or repeated* collection, analysis, and interpretation of health-related data and the dissemination of *information* to monitor the *health of a [human] population* and to identify potential risks to health, thereby enabling timely interventions to prevent, treat, or control disease and injury. It includes *occupational and environmental health surveillance and medical surveillance*

Comprehensive health surveillance (DoDD 6490.02E, 2012)

> Health surveillance conducted *throughout Service members' military careers* and DoD civilian employees' employment, across all duty locations, and encompassing risk, intervention, and outcome data. Such surveillance is essential to the evaluation, planning, and implementation of public health practice and

prevention and must be closely integrated with the ***timely dissemination of information*** to those who can ***act upon it.***

Medical surveillance (DoDD 6490.02E, 2012; Joint Publication 1-02, 2013)

The ongoing systematic collection, analysis, and interpretation of data derived from instances of medical care or medical evaluation, and the reporting of population-based information for characterizing and countering threats to a population's health, well-being, and performance.

Medical intelligence (DoDI 6420.01, 2009)

The product of collection, evaluation, and ***all-source analysis*** of ***worldwide health threats and issues***, including foreign medical capabilities, infectious disease, environmental health risks, developments in biotechnology and biomedical subjects of national and military importance, and ***support to force protection***.

DoD Documents Identify Different Levels of Missions Relevant to Biosurveillance

- **DoD mission:** provide the military forces needed to deter war and to protect the security of the United States
- **Goals**
    - Fit force, medically ready
    - Threat reduction
- **Strategic missions**
    - Force health protection
    - Global health security
    - Biological weapons defense
- **Lines of effort -- Operational missions**
    - Public health and medical care
    - International collaboration and capacity/capability building
    - Countering weapons of mass destruction
    - Health surveillance
    - Biosurveillance
    - R&D
    - Medical intelligence

The study team reviewed the approximately 30 DoD documents provided by AFHSC and identified and reviewed nearly 40 additional DoD documents related to biosurveillance and extracted each mention of "mission." The missions listed here are relevant directly or indirectly to biosurveillance, at different levels. The team organized these by tiers they created, to differentiate from the highest-level goals and strategic-level missions to lines of effort, or operational-level missions. Appendix B summarizes the specific sources for, and text related to, these missions.

The mission most directly related to biosurveillance is force health protection, which is defined as "measures to promote, improve, or conserve the behavioral and physical well-being of Service members to enable a healthy and fit force, prevent injury and illness, and protect the force from health hazards" (Joint Publication 1-02, 2013). Force health protection is vital to ensuring the DoD's overall mission to provide the military forces needed to deter war and to protect the security of the United States (DoD, 2012a).

The Study Team Developed Criteria to Prioritize Strategic Missions

Attributes	Criteria
Statutory authority	• Whether Congress has authorized the mission within the DoD • Whether there is a relevant legally binding obligation (e.g., international law)
National policy	• Whether there is either an explicit or implicit mission in a national policy/strategy or guidance document
DoD authority	• Whether DoD doctrine/policy defines mission • Whether the mission has been assigned to an Undersecretary or Assistant Secretary of Defense

OMB asked for a prioritization of missions relative to the DoD biosurveillance enterprise, so the study team developed criteria to help prioritize such missions. These are shown in the table and reflect criteria in descending order of importance. The team consulted authoritative sources (e.g., Congressional legislation, national policies, DoD authorities) to document the extent to which these criteria are fulfilled by DoD biosurveillance programs that address potentially important strategic missions.

Because statutory authorities underpin what DoD is and is not allowed to do, the team first searched for and examined the law to determine which missions are authorized by statute. Second, they identified relevant national policy documents (especially policy issued by the President), which can be directive for the U.S. government, although not inherently enshrined in Congressional legislation. Finally, they identified and examined internal DoD doctrine and policy documents.

The Three Strategic Missions Have Different Authorities

Mission	Statutory authorization of, or legal obligation for, mission	National policy that defines mission	DoD doctrine authorization of mission
Force health protection	Title 10 Chapter 55	None needed	• DoDD 6200.04 • ASD(HA) lead
Biological weapons defense	Title 50 Chapter 36	National Strategy for Countering Biological Threats	• DoDD 5160.05E • DoDD 5105.62 • USD(AT&L) lead
Global health security	WHO International Health Regulations (2005)	• Presidential Policy Directive National Science and Technology Council-7 • National Strategy for Biosurveillance • National Strategy for Countering Biological Threats • National Health Security Strategy • Global Health Security second-term agenda (White House, 6/27/13)	None

The study team found that there is clear statutory language as well as associated DoD doctrine that direct DoD to conduct the missions of force health protection and biological weapons defense, but neither statutory language nor DoD doctrine exists for global health security. However, budget guidance for fiscal year 2015, issued by the White House on June 27, 2013, specifies priorities related to the National Strategy for Countering Biological Threats and the associated Global Health Security second-term agenda. Specifically, it asks federal agencies, including DoD, to align relevant parts of their fiscal year 2015 budget requests with eight priority objectives under larger aims to (a) prevent avoidable epidemics, (b) detect threats early, and (c) respond rapidly and effectively. This issuance underscores the priority that the White House attaches to a U.S. global health security mission.

Also related to the global health security mission, the United States is a signatory to the WHO IHR, which is an international treaty that carries the force of international law. However, Congress has never explicitly authorized DoD to conduct this mission nor has it provided a funding stream for it. The most definitive explicit authorization for DoD comes from PDD NSTC-7 from 1996 (PDD NSTC-7, 1996), which, *inter alia,* calls upon DoD to expand its role in the support of a U.S. government global emerging infectious disease agenda that includes biosurveillance. The National Strategy for Biosurveillance (2012) and the National Health Security Strategy (2009) are both national-level policies—the first issued by the White House and the second by the Secretary of the Department of Health and Human Services (HHS)— which define a global health security mission for the Nation, though not explicitly for specific federal departments. Other than NSTC-7, no other policy directive authorizes a DoD global health security mission, although clearly it is an important mission given the wide dispersion of forces, the amount of global travel and trade that increase the spread of and vulnerability to epidemics (Moore, 2012), and the increasing threat posed by biological weapons.

Based on the strength of official authority, the study team determined that the most important mission relative to a biosurveillance capability is force health protection, followed by biological weapons defense, which is Congressionally mandated and also supports force health protection. Finally, global and more recent national policies point to the global health security mission as another critically important DoD mission, but yet to be mandated officially by U.S. statute and/or DoD doctrine/policy. The June 27, 2013, budget guidance from the White House addresses all relevant federal agencies, including DoD, and specifies priorities related to global health security with which these agencies should align relevant programs in their fiscal year 2015 budgets. Future Congressional appropriations to DoD that are explicit about global health security would be the first statutory authority to DoD in this area.

DoD has other missions that the team determined are not sufficiently related to biosurveillance to be included in this report. One example is Defense Support to Civil Authorities, which is authorized under the Stafford Act and DoD doctrine (42 U.S.C. 5121 et seq. Chapter 68; DoDD 3025.18, 2010) and fundamentally authorizes DoD military response action within the United States under specified emergency conditions.

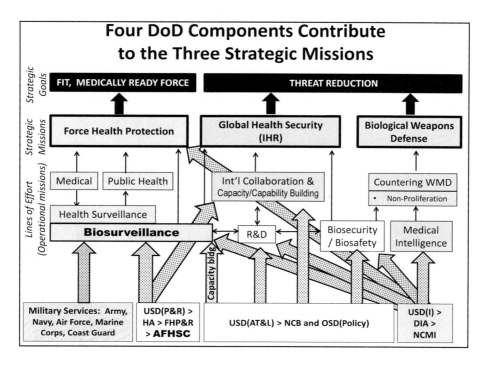

The capabilities and systems of the military Services and three OSD-level organizations comprise the DoD biosurveillance enterprise. The primary mission of each is as follows:

- Military Services: Organize, equip, and train forces
- AFHSC: Force health protection
- ASD(NCB): Biological weapons defense
- NCMI: Intelligence analysis of foreign medical capabilities and infectious disease threats for deployed forces.

Organizing the roles and responsibilities of each of these four main DoD actors based on strategic missions and lines of effort (operational-level missions) for each key actor reveals considerable overlap, in terms of the entities contributing to biosurveillance and to other strategic and operational DoD missions.

Specifically, the DoD biosurveillance enterprise encompasses the following activities:

- The biosurveillance, health surveillance, medical, and public health lines of effort (operational-level missions) carried out by the Services and AFHSC support the strategic force health protection mission (the U.S. Coast Guard, one of the military Services, is also included within DoD biosurveillance).
- The host nation biosurveillance capacity/capability building line of effort (operational-level mission) is conducted under the auspices of the ASD(NCB) and its subordinate organization, the Defense Threat Reduction Agency (DTRA) through CBEP, as well as by AFHSC's GEIS, and supports a strategic global health security mission (these efforts are fully consistent with the provisions and obligations of the U.S. government and other developed countries, under the WHO's IHR.
- The biosecurity/biosafety, medical intelligence, and countering weapons of mass destruction lines of effort (operational-level missions) carried out by DTRA, the ASD(NCB), and NCMI support a strategic biological weapons defense mission.

AFHSC is the designated coordinator of DoD "health surveillance" and "comprehensive health surveillance" (DoDD 6490.02E, 2012), which monitor human health (including environmental health) risks and events in military and affiliated populations.

Several programs fall under the Under Secretary of Defense for Acquisitions, Technology and Logistics (USD[AT&L]). For example, the Joint Program Executive Office is the department's focal point for research, development, acquisition, fielding, and long-term support of biological defense equipment and medical countermeasures. The considerable surveillance effort that deals with biological weapons defense is under the direction of the ASD(NCB) and focuses on four main areas: medical countermeasures, diagnostics, biosurveillance, and non-traditional agent defense. Programs include advancing technology for early warning and detection of threats, countermeasure development, creating data communication and analysis platforms, and improving personal protective equipment. Finally, the origins of the CBEP focused exclusively on the Former Soviet Union and date back to the early post–Cold War period. The program still maintains a focus on "especially dangerous pathogens" even as it expands to other countries and regions.

Medical intelligence is an important and unique DoD effort. It is a good example of a central DoD program that is otherwise non-traditional in the civilian biosurveillance world. The DoD biosurveillance enterprise draws from the Intelligence Community to include an "early warning" component that utilizes intelligence tradecraft to identify and forecast emerging potentially destabilizing biological threats. Medical intelligence activities are carried out by NCMI, which falls under the DIA.

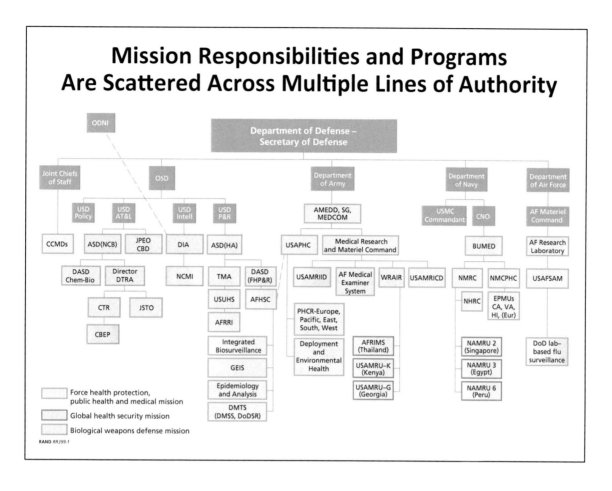

Mission Responsibilities and Programs Are Scattered Across Multiple Lines of Authority

RAND RR399-1

Showing these organizational entities and their missions based on DoD's organizational structure indicates even more clearly how similar missions are managed across different military lines of authority.

AFHSC is managed as an Executive Agency under the Army, with its operational funding through the U.S. Army Public Health Command (USAPHC). However, it receives functional direction from the Deputy Assistant Secretary of Defense for Force Health Protection and Readiness (DASD[FHP&R]), who reports to the Assistant Secretary of Defense for Health Affairs (ASD[HA]). AFHSC's own operational funding is routed through the Department of the Army chain of command (shown as dotted line); funding within AFHSC's GEIS budget for CONUS and OCONUS laboratories is routed directly through the relevant Services. ASD(NCB) also provides some funding to OCONUS laboratories.

NCMI is shown within DoD under the Under Secretary of Defense (Intelligence), but its authority and funding are from the Intelligence Community, specifically the Office of the Director of National Intelligence (also shown as dotted line in the figure).

The CCMDs and the Services, focused primarily on achieving force health protection goals, have a significant investment in biosurveillance in that they conduct continuous monitoring of U.S. forces' health across the globe. Also, to some degree the CCMD efforts in biological weapons defense are aimed at protecting the health of the force.

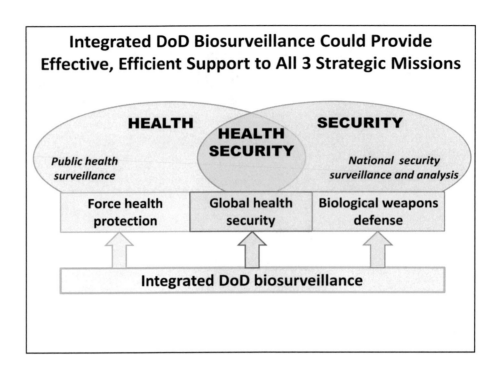

Integrated DoD Biosurveillance Could Provide Effective, Efficient Support to All 3 Strategic Missions

Well-integrated DoD biosurveillance could provide effective, efficient, and important support to all three relevant DoD strategic missions. These missions are, in turn, consistent with higher-level national health, health security, and security policy.

Identification of Biosurveillance Programs and Assets

DoD Supports Many Biosurveillance-Related Systems and Assets

- **Biosurveillance systems for military and affiliated populations**
  - Reportable medical events
  - Outbreaks of defined syndromes
  - Deployment health assessments
  - Medical encounters (CONUS, OCONUS), with or without associated lab tests, pharmacy transactions
  - Individual Medical Readiness indicators (e.g., immunizations)
  - Occupational and environmental health readiness
- **Collaborative biosurveillance in other countries**
  - Collaborative surveillance for emerging infections and biosurveillance capacity / capability building for host countries' situational awareness and reporting
  - Outbreaks of defined syndromes
  - Cooperative research studies (with host nation) on human and animal disease caused by "especially dangerous pathogens"
- **Biosurveillance assets**
  - Laboratories (CONUS, OCONUS; point of care → reference level)
  - DoD Serum Repository
  - Infrastructure building programs (e.g., lab construction, training, information technology systems)
  - Medical intelligence capabilities and products

AFHSC provided the study team with a comprehensive list of DoD organizations with programming relevant to biosurveillance, including R&D organizations and programs. The list specified the owner, purpose, data stream, and frequency of each effort. The study team selected those that reflected biosurveillance system processes or assets (i.e., consciously omitting R&D programs).

The foundation of the DoD biosurveillance enterprise is comprised of multiple programs that draw upon information technology and laboratory assets. Some of these monitor the health and environment related to military and affiliated populations, including

- reportable medical events (n=66, including 63 specific diseases or pathogens)
- outbreaks of defined syndromes
- pre- and post-deployment health assessments and reassessments
- medical encounters in CONUS and OCONUS, with or without laboratory and other diagnostic test results and pharmacy transactions
- Individual Medical Readiness indicators (e.g., immunizations)
- occupational and environmental health readiness.

Other programs help partner countries build their capacity and capabilities and monitor biological events in their populations, such as outbreaks of defined syndromes.

Additional assets include the network of Army (Thailand, Kenya, Georgia) and Navy (Egypt, Singapore, Peru) OCONUS laboratories; Service and other CONUS-based clinical diagnostic and reference laboratories; the DoD Serum Repository, which now includes over 55 million serum specimens collected longitudinally over the careers of Service members; infrastructure building programs that, for example, help build laboratories and train laboratory technicians and epidemiologists; and medical intelligence assets that provide finished intelligence products related to endemic and epidemic diseases and the capabilities of foreign medical systems worldwide.

Each System Serves at Least One Strategic Mission

Biosurveillance system or asset Strategic Mission →	FHP	BWD	GHS
Acute Respiratory Disease Surveillance System	X		
Army and Navy OCONUS laboratories	X	*	X
Casualty data (Armed Forces Medical Examiners System)	X		
Cooperative Biological Engagement Program (CBEP) – capacity building			X
Defense Health Services Systems (DHSS)	X		
Defense Medical Surveillance System (DMSS)	X		
Defense Occupational and Environmental Health Readiness System (DOEHRS)	X		
Deployment health assessments (5 Services)	X		
DoD Serum Repository	X		
Early Warning Outbreak Response System (EWORS – Asia)			X
Electronic Surveillance System for Early Notification of Community-based Epidemics (ESSENCE)	X		
Embassy-based respiratory surveillance			X
Global DoD lab-based Influenza Surveillance and Response System (Air Force)	X		X
Global Emerging Infections Surveillance and Response System (GEIS)	X		X
Joint Biological Agent Identification and Diagnostic System (JBAIDS)		X	
Medical Situational Awareness in Theater (MSAT)	X		
National Center for Medical Intelligence (NCMI)	X	X	X
Reportable medical events (5 Services)	X		
Suite for Automated Global Electronic bioSurveillance (SAGES)			X
U.S. Army Research Institute of Infectious Disease (USAMRIID)	X	X	

* Based on government grants

The study team identified approximately 30 military biosurveillance systems and assets, including laboratories, characterized them based on the strategic-level mission(s) served, and then added details related to selected performance criteria (the table above presents examples, characterized by mission; see Appendix C for full listing and the associated performance characteristics, which are described further in Chapter Three).

Desired Outcomes

The National Strategy for Biosurveillance Suggests Desired Outcomes from DoD Biosurveillance

- Definition of biosurveillance
  - "...the process of gathering, integrating, interpreting, and communicating essential information related to all-hazards threats or disease activity affecting human, animal, or plant health to achieve **early detection and warning**, contribute to overall **situational awareness** of the health aspects of an incident, and to enable **better decisionmaking** at all levels."

- Of four key functions, one is:
  - "**forecast** and advise impacts"

The National Strategy for Biosurveillance suggests desired outcomes from biosurveillance:

- Early warning of threats and early detection of events
- Overall situational awareness
- Better decision making at all levels
- Forecast of impacts.

The "Joint DOTmLPF-P Change Recommendation for Biosurveillance" (JROCM 116-13, dated June 6, 2013) notes two main functions "required for robust, responsive DoD biosurveillance capability" (Joint Staff/J-8, 2013), which are consistent with the desired outcomes noted above:

- Rapid detection, identification, analysis (including characterization), and impact assessment related to diagnosis of disease or pathogens or to health hazards
- Timely reporting and early warning of results and related information to those responsible for decisions and actions

Moreover, numerous other DoD and non-DoD sources validate these outcomes (DoDD 6490.02E, 2012; DoDD 6200.04, 2007; HSPD 21, 2007; CDC, 2001; Institute of Medicine, 2002; CDC, 2010; Thacker, 2000; WHO, 2008).

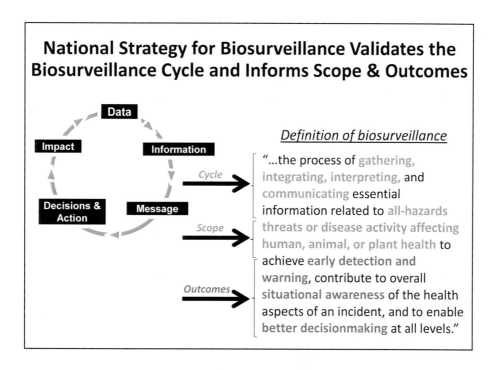

National Strategy for Biosurveillance Validates the Biosurveillance Cycle and Informs Scope & Outcomes

Definition of biosurveillance

"...the process of gathering, integrating, interpreting, and communicating essential information related to all-hazards threats or disease activity affecting human, animal, or plant health to achieve early detection and warning, contribute to overall situational awareness of the health aspects of an incident, and to enable better decisionmaking at all levels."

The public health surveillance cycle is a process that transforms data into information and messages that can then reach decision makers for decisions and actions (McNabb, 2002; Moore, 2012; Nsubuga, 2006) The process will only have impact if data are transformed in this way into understandable, actionable information and are communicated to those who need to know (Nsubuga, 2006). The transformation of "data" into "information" (i.e., data that are interpreted and presented in a way decision makers understand clearly and can act upon) is particularly relevant within the military, where some decision makers—such as combatant commanders—typically are not health professionals. Such interpretation is often left to the public health professionals working under the CCMD surgeons, who must take data and multiple reports and interpret them in a way that facilitates decision making by their commanders.

The National Strategy for Biosurveillance validates the public health surveillance cycle: The definition of biosurveillance includes the gathering, integrating, interpreting, and communicating of essential information, to enable decision making at all levels. The Strategy also informs the scope of biosurveillance to include all-hazards threats that affect human, animal or plant health. Finally, the definition offers three of the four desired outcomes of biosurveillance, with the fourth coming from one of the four key functions in the Strategy.

Performance Measures and Targets

Several Approaches Can Inform Development of a Package of Biosurveillance Performance Measures

- Parameters suggested by AFHSC CONOPS plan
- Lessons from "performance-based accountability systems"
- Lessons from development of CDC's public health emergency preparedness capabilities and associated measures
- Criteria used for assessment of civilian surveillance system performance
- Measures developed based on strategic plans of key DoD actors (e.g., AFHSC strategic plan)
- Measures suggested by 2013 internal DoD working group
- Measures currently under development by Interagency Policy Committee for Global Health Security
- Consideration of relevant existing measures (e.g., from CDC, Healthy People 2020, U.S. government's IHR core capacity measures)

Performance measurement is fundamentally about monitoring and evaluation to document progress and inform changes to improve programs—ultimately, to improve program outcomes and impacts. Performance measures can reflect inputs, actions, outputs, or outcomes.

The AFHSC concept of operations (CONOPS) (2009) specifies that performance measures should be identified from appropriate national sources and additional ones developed as needed (AFHSC, 2009). Sections 11.1–11.4 specifically call for

- "a variety of structure, process, and outcome measures [that] will best facilitate process improvement"
- monitoring across the entire DoD biosurveillance enterprise
- consideration of the Military Health System Strategic Plan
- consideration of criteria that "include relevance, feasibility, actionability, reliability, and validity."

There are different approaches to consider in developing performance measures for the DoD biosurveillance enterprise. All are relatively time- and labor-intensive if they are done properly. Therefore, this report does not purport to have a comprehensive set of measures, but rather, offers insights and some examples of approaches and measures that can be considered as part of an appropriate DoD performance measure development process.

Since the 1990s, performance measurement within the context of performance-based accountability systems has become more popular among public policy makers; such systems link incentives (financial or other; positive or negative) to measured performance as a way to improve services. A 2010 study by the RAND Corporation examined nine public sector examples from five sectors, including health (Camm, 2010). It found the approach promising but the evidence base for its effectiveness still limited. Nonetheless, several key findings are relevant to consideration of DoD biosurveillance performance measurement:

- Key components include goals, incentives, and performance measures that are well-defined and widely shared among all key stakeholders.
- Tensions exist between selection of existing (available) measures and optimal measures that may not yet exist, and between measures of short-term outputs versus longer-term outcomes and impact, for accountability purposes.
- Performance measures should matter: measures that actors can influence, are easily observable and unambiguous, and are meaningful to key stakeholders

To the extent that DoD biosurveillance is relevant to analogous activity in the civilian sector, the CDC's recent experience in working with partners to develop measures for public health emergency preparedness capabilities also offers insights for development of biosurveillance measures for DoD (Shelton, 2013). Key lessons derived from that experience included the following:

- Identify intended users and uses: Examples of main uses included accountability (e.g., making funding decisions), performance management and quality improvement (e.g., deriving lessons and best practices), and research (e.g., understanding determinants and variation in measurement data). The different categories of use are typically aimed at different users, from external to internal stakeholders.
- Determine what should be measured: Reviewing existing measures and the evidence base for them, eliciting inputs from practitioners and other key stakeholders, and analyzing the processes encompassed by the envisaged measures.
- Ensure data quality: Availability of data and feasibility of collection, selection of data for which variability is relevant to performance (reducing irrelevant variation), and clarifying key definitions.
- Assess utility and acceptability of measures through consultation and pilot testing.

The National Strategy for Biosurveillance does not include performance measures. However, the CDC and a more recent study by Moore et al. have suggested criteria for assessing surveillance system performance (CDC, 2001; Moore et al., 2008). The study team adapted these criteria for use in the present assessment, as described in Chapter Three. They can be considered as part of an overall "performance measurement package" for DoD biosurveillance:

- Coverage/completeness
- Quality/accuracy
- Timeliness
- Integration

Another way to organize performance measurement could be derived from AFHSC's Strategic Plan for fiscal years 2013–2015 (AFHSC, 2013a), with additions to reflect similar-level planning for other key DoD actors such as ASD(NCB) and NCMI. The AFHSC plan includes six strategic goals, each with specified sub-goals and performance objectives. Some performance objectives reflect actions toward desired end states, while others reflect actions to improve inputs, processes, outputs, and customer orientation. Some objectives appear to lend themselves to development of corresponding performance measures, recognizing that they cover a broad range—from inputs to processes, outputs, and outcomes. DoD can consider whether and how to narrow the focus for measurement purposes.

Yet another approach to biosurveillance metrics is reflected in a May 2013 internal working paper developed by the Defense Health Agency (DHA) Sub-Working Group on Public Health (DHA Public Health sub Work Group, 2013). That document suggests seven "functional metrics" that focus on "process improvement and elimination of redundancy" in DoD health surveillance. While likely useful as part of a larger package of DoD biosurveillance performance measures, these appear to be relatively narrow in terms of the overall DoD biosurveillance enterprise, for which appropriate performance measures might also importantly relate to data systems and processes, outputs, outcomes, and mission impact.

At the time of this report, the Interagency Policy Committee for Global Health Security was working to finalize measures to support the Global Health Security second-term agenda specified in the White House guidance issued on June 27, 2013. These measures, once finalized officially, may be especially relevant to DoD's biosurveillance performance monitoring.

Finally, a number of existing measures from outside DoD merit consideration as DoD undertakes a systematic effort to develop performance measures and standards for its overall biosurveillance enterprise. Some illustrative examples are shown in Table 2.1.

Table 2.1. Illustrative Examples of Existing Performance Measures

Source	Measure
Public Health Preparedness Capabilities (CDC) (CDC, 2011)	Proportion of reports of selected reportable diseases received within the required time frame
	Proportion of reports of selected reportable disease for which initial public health control measure(s) were initiated within the appropriate time frame
	Percentage of [specified] proficiency tests successfully passed by [specified laboratories]
	Time for [specified laboratories] to notify [specified DoD authorities and other public health partners] of significant laboratory results
	Percentage of clinical specimens without any adverse quality assurance events received at the [specified central laboratory] for confirmation or rule-out testing from clinical laboratories
	Ability of the [specified laboratories] to collect relevant samples for clinical analysis, packaging, and shipment of those samples
Healthy People 2020 Public Health Infrastructure (PHI) objective (HHS. Office of Disease Prevention and Health Promotion)	Proportion of [specified DoD] laboratories that provide or assure comprehensive laboratory services to support essential public health services 1. Disease prevention, control and surveillance (PHI-11.1) 2. Integrated data management (PHI-11.2) 3. Reference and specialized testing (PHI-11.3) 4. Emergency response (PHI-11.8)
U.S. government measures for IHR core capacity development(Ijaz et al., 2012; White House National Security Staff, 2011)	Human resources: Number of trained field epidemiologists per 200,000 population (target: at least one)
	Laboratory: Countries have access to the capacity to reliably conduct core diagnostic tests on specimens obtained and transported from any part of the country (target: ten such tests, including six specified tests and four as specified by a country based on relevance)
	Syndrome detection: Country's system demonstrates the ability to detect syndromes indicative of a potential public health emergency of international concern using international reference quality standards for these syndromic surveillance systems (target: at least three of the five specified syndromes)
	Rapid response teams: Number of rostered, trained, and drilled rapid response teams capable of responding to an infectious disease outbreak within 24 hours of its identification (target: at least one per administrative unit [state, province, department, or other with population size 10,000–100,000])

Key Findings

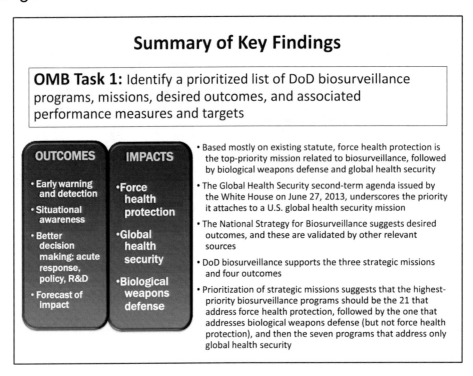

The first task from the OMB was to "identify a prioritized list of DoD biosurveillance programs, missions, desired outcomes, and associated performance measures and targets" to track progress toward achieving those outcomes. Because the DoD biosurveillance enterprise is not comprised of a single program, the study team examined the DoD strategic missions to which the biosurveillance enterprise contributes and prioritized those missions.

Based on review of U.S. statute and international law, national policy, DoD doctrine/policy, and funded DoD programs, the team determined that the highest-priority strategic DoD mission relevant to biosurveillance is force health protection, followed by biological weapons defense (which itself also supports force health protection). Recent national policy documents and the internationally binding WHO IHR justify a third strategic-level DoD mission—global health security. Important DoD programming, including programming supported by U.S statute, contributes to global health security.

The National Strategy for Biosurveillance, issued in July 2012, suggests desired outcomes for biosurveillance. These are relevant to DoD biosurveillance as well:

- Early warning of threats and early detection of events
- Situational awareness
- Better decision making at all levels, including acute response, policy, and R&D
- Forecast of impacts.

DoD biosurveillance supports the three strategic-level missions and four desired outcomes:

- NCMI in particular provides indicators and early warning and forecasting of impact

34

- AFHSC/GEIS, NCMI, and CBEP all contribute to situational awareness globally, and Service and AFHSC biosurveillance support situational awareness among military Service members
- All components of the DoD biosurveillance enterprise enable decision making by DoD, the U.S. government, and host nation officials

Biosurveillance programs can in turn be prioritized based on the relative priority of these three strategic-level missions, with programs supporting force health protection accorded the highest priority.

Performance measures can monitor relevant inputs, actions, outputs, and outcomes. Development of performance measures and targets typically requires intensive efforts over months or years; the study team identified a number of potentially relevant measures that can be considered.

3. OMB Task 2—Performance

OMB Task 2: Evaluate how the current array of program assets contributes to achieving the prioritized missions

Findings:

- High coverage and quality, especially for service members
- Potential for more-frequent data analysis and more-robust integration
- Potential for enhanced mission achievement through

    - new DoD doctrine/policy, governance, and organization (DHA)
    - increased AFHSC/DIB staffing
    - better AFHSC physical infrastructure (classified terminals and computing facility for access to classified information; possibly an operations center for near-real-time monitoring)

Methods

OMB Task 2: Evaluate how the current array of program assets contributes to achieving the prioritized missions

- Define and apply criteria to assess the performance of DoD biosurveillance systems and assets (<u>processes</u>)

    - Characterize systems and assets according to these criteria

    - Apply the criteria to assess performance

- Define and apply criteria to assess <u>inputs</u>—enabling functions that support DoD biosurveillance

- Define and apply criteria to assess DoD biosurveillance <u>outputs</u>

    - Identify and examine biosurveillance products (outputs)

    - Apply the criteria to assess outputs

The second task from OMB was to evaluate how the current array of program assets contributes to achieving the prioritized missions. To address this task, the study team defined and applied criteria to assess performance of DoD biosurveillance systems and assets, drawing from relevant published guidance and other sources. The team characterized DoD biosurveillance systems and assets according to these criteria and applied the criteria to assess performance. They then defined and applied criteria to assess inputs – enabling functions that support DoD biosurveillance, using a DOTMLPF-like structure (doctrine, organization, training, materiel, leadership and education, personnel, and facilities). Finally, they defined and applied criteria to assess DoD biosurveillance outputs.

The Study Team Developed Criteria to Assess Processes – Biosurveillance Programs and Assets

System Attributes	Criteria
(1) Coverage / Completeness	• Wide range of locations, sources, populations, pathogens or conditions monitored, clinical data streams • Appropriately large size, representative distribution of populations
(2) Quality / Accuracy	• Data are standardized • Accurate diagnosis: lab-confirmed > clinical > "pre-clinical" self-report • Lab testing is included and accurate: genetic sequencing > characterization > identification > screening > none
(3) Timeliness	• Appropriate frequency of collection, transmission, analysis, communication • Near-real-time (daily) capability, if warranted, otherwise, timeliness appropriate to potential action
(4) Integration	• Whether data system is linked to (i.e., received by) AFHSC, and into which data system (e.g., DMSS, GEIS, other) • Format of data • Links to other relevant data streams • Integrated across military Services • Linked beyond DoD

Source: Adapted from Moore et al., 2008; and CDC 2001

The CDC has provided guidance for assessing public health surveillance system performance (CDC, 2001). More recently, Moore et al. condensed the assessment domains into a smaller number relevant to global influenza surveillance and also relevant for assessing DoD biosurveillance (Moore et al., 2008). Because of the focus of this study and the evolving priorities of biosurveillance more generally, the study team added a new criterion related to integration. The four major criteria used to characterize and assess each relevant DoD biosurveillance system or asset were

- Coverage/Completeness: Refers to the range of locations, sources, populations, pathogens or conditions monitored, and clinical data streams, as well as the size and distribution of populations monitored.
- Quality/Accuracy: Refers to standardization of data, accuracy of diagnosis (laboratory-confirmed is more accurate than clinical diagnosis, which in turn is more accurate than "pre-clinical" chief complaint or self-report), and the inclusion and accuracy of laboratory testing (genetic sequencing provides the most granular level of detail, followed by laboratory characterization, identification, or screening).
- Timeliness: Refers to the frequency of data collection, transmission, analysis, and communication, ranging from near-real-time (typically considered as daily) to weekly, monthly, quarterly, or annual.
- Integration: Refers to both internal and external linkages—whether the data system is linked to (i.e., received by) a central DoD entity such as AFHSC—the format of the data (standardized/interoperable or not), whether the data are linked to other relevant data streams and/or across military Services, and whether data/information is also drawn from systems beyond DoD (e.g., CDC, Department of Homeland Security [DHS], WHO) and integrated into DoD's analyses for situational awareness or other purposes.

The team characterized each of the approximately 30 biosurveillance programs (systems and assets) according to these criteria (see Appendix C), based on information gleaned from document review and internet searches. AFHSC staff graciously helped provide missing information, especially related to frequency of data collection, transmission, and analysis, but also other features for which documentation available to the study team was incomplete.

(1a) Population Coverage: Biosurveillance Coverage in Military Populations Is Comprehensive

- Biosurveillance in military Service members and affiliated populations supports the force health protection mission

- Health surveillance includes monitoring of all DoD Service members throughout their careers

- Surveillance also includes military-affiliated populations
  - Dependents residing in garrisons or based overseas
  - Military civilians deployed overseas

The first attribute assessed is coverage/completeness, beginning with population coverage, which refers to the percentage of populations that are monitored.

Population coverage of U.S. military members is comprehensive—in principle essentially universal. This strongly supports DoD's and AFHSC's force health protection mission.

Biosurveillance also covers certain military-affiliated populations, including military dependents, and deployed military civilians. Coverage of these populations also supports the force health protection mission.

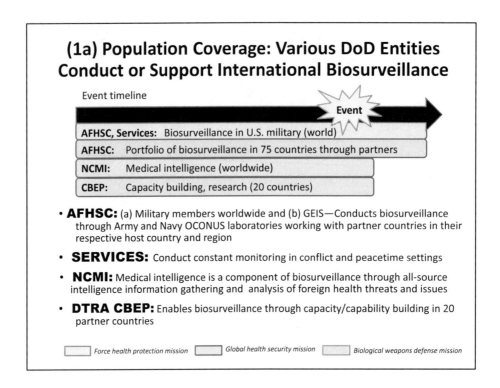

(1a) Population Coverage: Various DoD Entities Conduct or Support International Biosurveillance

Event timeline

Event

AFHSC, Services: Biosurveillance in U.S. military (world)

AFHSC: Portfolio of biosurveillance in 75 countries through partners

NCMI: Medical intelligence (worldwide)

CBEP: Capacity building, research (20 countries)

- **AFHSC:** (a) Military members worldwide and (b) GEIS—Conducts biosurveillance through Army and Navy OCONUS laboratories working with partner countries in their respective host country and region

- **SERVICES:** Conduct constant monitoring in conflict and peacetime settings

- **NCMI:** Medical intelligence is a component of biosurveillance through all-source intelligence information gathering and analysis of foreign health threats and issues

- **DTRA CBEP:** Enables biosurveillance through capacity/capability building in 20 partner countries

Force health protection mission   *Global health security mission*   *Biological weapons defense mission*

Biosurveillance entails monitoring of health-related information before an event, detection of the event, and in some instances monitoring after an event has occurred (e.g., for ongoing situational awareness). Various DoD entities conduct or support international biosurveillance. This includes surveillance of U.S. military members based or deployed worldwide, in support of the force health protection mission. As noted previously, surveillance coverage among military members is essentially universal (nearly 100-percent population coverage).

For biosurveillance in foreign populations, the AFHSC houses, supports, and coordinates GEIS. Army and Navy OCONUS laboratories are major GEIS participants, providing the epidemiological and laboratory support to selected countries in the laboratories' areas of responsibility. The Cooperative Threat Reduction (CTR) program within the DTRA supports the CBEP, which includes biosurveillance as one program objective. CBEP enables biosurveillance by supporting capacity/capabilities building and cooperative biological research. CBEP documentation indicates that the program is active in 20 countries in the Former Soviet Union, South and Southeast Asia, Afghanistan, Iraq, and Africa (full list found in Appendix C, Table C.2).

NCMI produces finished medical intelligence products on endemic and epidemic diseases and health/medical care systems in countries worldwide.

Population coverage for biosurveillance in foreign populations is the purview of each partner country, i.e., in conducting its own public health surveillance. DoD assistance to strengthen the capacity and capabilities of those countries supports a global health security mission. Population coverage is inherently less complete compared to coverage among military Service members. However, less than full population coverage is typical of traditional public health surveillance.

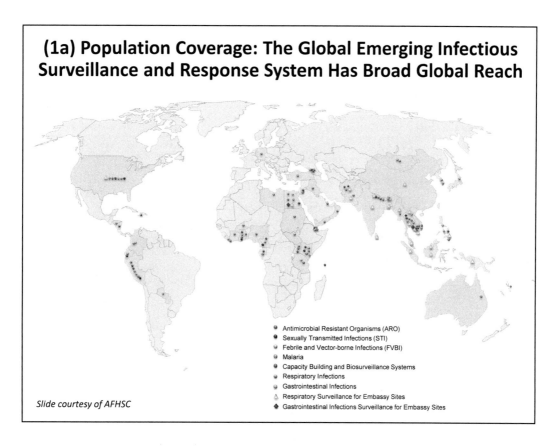

(1a) Population Coverage: The Global Emerging Infectious Surveillance and Response System Has Broad Global Reach

Slide courtesy of AFHSC

- ⬤ Antimicrobial Resistant Organisms (ARO)
- ⬤ Sexually Transmitted Infections (STI)
- ⬤ Febrile and Vector-borne Infections (FVBI)
- ⬤ Malaria
- ⬤ Capacity Building and Biosurveillance Systems
- ⬤ Respiratory Infections
- ⬤ Gastrointestinal Infections
- △ Respiratory Surveillance for Embassy Sites
- ◆ Gastrointestinal Infections Surveillance for Embassy Sites

In fiscal year 2013, GEIS funded 33 distinct DoD and non-DoD partners and supported a network of approximately 75 countries in U.S. Africa Command (22 countries), U.S. Central Command (10 countries), U.S. European Command (9 countries), U.S. Pacific Command (22 countries), and U.S. Southern Command (12 countries), as shown in the map above and detailed in Appendix D.

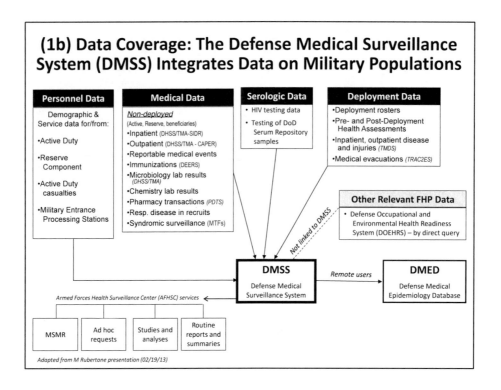

(1b) Data Coverage: The Defense Medical Surveillance System (DMSS) Integrates Data on Military Populations

Adapted from M Rubertone presentation (02/19/13)

The second dimension of biosurveillance coverage/completeness is data coverage, referring to the breadth of diseases/conditions monitored and associated variables.

Data coverage for military Service members is very robust, just as for population coverage among them.

The Defense Medical Surveillance System (DMSS), created and maintained by AFHSC, is a unique military database that captures a broad range of data streams relevant to the health of military populations across their years of military service. This is a relational database that enables a robust range of epidemiological analysis. It is the only military database linked to the DoD Serum Repository. Details of data feeds into DMSS as of March 2013 are shown in Appendix E.

The principal military health surveillance asset not linked through DMSS is the Defense Occupational and Environmental Health Readiness System (DOEHRS), which must be queried separately to assess environmental health risks.

(1b) Data Coverage: International Biosurveillance Data Are Robust but Selective

- **GEIS collaborates with partner countries to support their surveillance for five key syndromes**
  - Respiratory infections with an emphasis on avian and pandemic influenza
  - Gastrointestinal infections
  - Febrile and vector-borne infections
  - Antimicrobial resistance
  - Sexually transmitted infections
- **Other systems monitor selective diseases internationally**
  - Clusters of cases with respiratory symptoms in U.S. Embassy personnel in 46 countries
  - CBEP-supported laboratory and epidemiology capacity/capabilities building related to "especially dangerous pathogens" (Group A Select agents and pathogens with pandemic potential); cooperative biological research studies include both human and animal diseases
  - Daily monitoring by NCMI of 70–80 diseases/pathogens of military relevance

Data coverage internationally—foreign governments' own surveillance and DoD surveillance in non-military U.S. embassy personnel in other countries—is robust but selective. Data cover a broad and relevant range of diseases and syndromes, but most data are aggregated rather than case-specific, which limits the range of possible analyses. Also, most DoD biosurveillance is in humans; however, through some CBEP-supported studies, foreign governments collect epidemiological data on animal diseases within their country.

GEIS collaborates with partner countries to support their surveillance for five key syndromes of interest to the countries and to DoD:

- respiratory infections, with an emphasis on avian and pandemic influenza
- gastrointestinal infections
- febrile and vector-borne infections
- antimicrobial resistance
- sexually-transmitted infections.

Other systems monitor selective diseases internationally:

- The Department of State, supported by the Walter Reed Army Institute of Research (WRAIR) and DoD OCONUS laboratories in Thailand, Kenya, and Peru, monitors clusters of cases with respiratory symptoms in U.S. Embassy personnel in 46 countries (see Table C.1 in Appendix C)
- CBEP helps countries build their laboratory and epidemiology capacity/capabilities related to "especially dangerous pathogens"—Group A Select Agents and pathogens with pandemic potential. This is the only component of the DoD biosurveillance enterprise that specifically supports collection of epidemiological data and laboratory testing for animal diseases.
- NCMI monitors daily 70–80 diseases/pathogens of military relevance and contextualizes analyses and forecasts that take into account a wide range of other data from all sources.

---

(2) Quality: DoD Biosurveillance Quality/Accuracy Is Generally High

- **Data quality in military Service members is generally high**
  - Analytical power of having denominator data to perform population surveillance analyses
  - Standardized case definitions (reportable medical events) and codes (clinical diagnoses)
  - High military standards for DoD clinical and reference laboratory and other testing (but possibly not as available in deployed field settings)
  - Serum Repository that can link biological specimens to biosurveillance data (high-quality material for antibody testing, but less reliable for testing that requires genetic material)
- **Data quality internationally is also relatively high**
  - High quality of laboratory diagnosis through OCONUS and CBEP-supported labs
  - Laboratory testing (screening through reference lab testing in some instances) for most biosurveillance for respiratory illness and dangerous pathogens
  - Less than definitive diagnosis for syndromic surveillance conducted by countries with GEIS support, unless laboratory testing is undertaken
  - To provide rapid warning of emerging health threats, NCMI's medical intelligence analysis is based on information that is preliminary and incomplete

---

The second dimension of biosurveillance system performance is quality or accuracy, referring to the inclusion of laboratory testing, the level of sophistication of the testing, and the reliability of reported clinical diagnoses or syndromes.

The quality of biosurveillance data in military Service members is generally high, for several reasons:

- The availability of denominator data greatly increases the analytical power of performing population surveillance analyses.
- Clinical diagnoses use standardized case definitions and clinical diagnostic codes.
- DoD clinical and reference laboratory and other testing meets high military standards (but may not be as available in deployed field settings).
- The Serum Repository is a resource that enables linkage of biological specimens with biosurveillance data (high-quality material for antibody testing, but less reliable for preservation of genetic material). (Moore et al., 2010)

However, AFHSC reports that these data are not validated; controls are in place to improve quality, but some data are missing and cannot be validated. Moreover, self-reports (e.g., pre- and post-deployment health assessments) may be of more questionable quality because they may not reflect the full extent of problems that Service members may consider stigmatizing, such as mental health problems.

The quality of international biosurveillance data populations is also relatively high, for several reasons:

- Laboratory diagnosis through OCONUS and CBEP-supported labs is typically very high quality.

- Most biosurveillance for respiratory illness or dangerous pathogens is supported by DoD definitive or reference lab testing. For example, testing for influenza often includes genetic sequencing of influenza viruses from samples collected through biosurveillance. Testing of dangerous pathogens is carried out by qualified CBEP-supported laboratories in partner countries and by the U.S. Army Medical Research Institute for Infectious Diseases (USAMRIID) and other DoD laboratories.
- Syndromic surveillance typically does not reflect definitive diagnosis, unless laboratory testing is undertaken.
- To provide rapid warning of emerging health threats, NCMI's medical intelligence analysis is based on information that is preliminary and incomplete. Intelligence warning is intended to drive mitigation of the threat's impact on U.S. forces.

The third dimension of biosurveillance system performance is timeliness, referring to the appropriateness of the frequency of data collection, data feeds to AFHSC and data analysis. These frequencies are captured for the ~30 systems and assets analyzed in this study (Tables C.1 and C.2 in Appendix C).

AFHSC typically analyzes biosurveillance data on military Service members weekly to monthly, quarterly, or annually. A CCMD with which the study team spoke noted the absence of near-real-time analysis that helps the CCMDs better understand the threats to the populations in their area of responsibility. While the AFHSC performs daily data analyses for some military Service member data (DMSS and theater medical encounters) this is to prepare reports that typically reflect historical trends, not current situational analysis. However, it does monitor interagency sources of information daily, for situational awareness purposes. The relative paucity of daily analysis and reporting based on near-real-time monitoring by AFHSC—for example, drawing upon DoD's Electronic Surveillance System for the Early Notification of Community-based Epidemics (ESSENCE) and other relevant near-real-time data—suggest that DoD biosurveillance may not detect and/or may not disseminate information about critical disease outbreaks or other conditions that might be time-sensitive. However, discussions with AFHSC indicated that AFHSC receives ad hoc reports of time-sensitive cases or outbreaks and is able to provide data in a timely way for policy purposes. A recent example is a case of an active duty Service member who recently returned from the Middle East with respiratory illness compatible with Middle East respiratory syndrome caused by the associated novel coronavirus (MERS—CoV). Early ad hoc notification by a GEIS partner lab to AFHSC enabled timely follow-up and investigation by AFHSC. This in turn informed timely decisions regarding protection of other active duty Service members who had traveled or will travel to the region or who had come into

48

contact with this individual. Similarly, public health surveillance in the civilian sector involves routine weekly reporting but also has mechanisms for reporting and responding to more time-sensitive outbreaks.

DoD could increase the frequency of its biosurveillance data analysis. For example, the Services collect health surveillance data on reportable medical events on a daily basis, but only send data to AFHSC weekly. AFHSC publishes weekly communicable disease reports (similar to the civilian CDC's weekly reporting). Occupational/environmental health data are available and can be queried as needed. The final operating capacity for AFHSC's Division of Integrated Biosurveillance (DIB) includes daily analysis and daily written reports, if resources become available. AFHSC noted that one reason for not performing more routine daily analysis for situational awareness purposes is the current manpower shortage. The final operating capability for the DIB includes more staff and plans for routine daily analyses for situational awareness purposes.

AFHSC's GEIS receives biosurveillance reports that partner countries choose to release, through the OCONUS laboratories and other GEIS partners. Such reports are typically sent less frequently and are thus less frequently available for analysis compared to biosurveillance data related to military populations. Only NCMI undertakes systematic daily examination of worldwide disease information. AFHSC's GEIS and the DIB might carefully consider whether and which global biosurveillance elements merit more frequent examination and dissemination of more timely reports, for situational awareness that supports both force health protection and global health security missions, and how data collected by partner countries might be made available for these purposes.

Finally, timeliness also includes the availability of technical information and support around the clock. From the perspective of the two CCMD public health professionals, it would be enormously helpful to have access to AFHSC technical support dedicated to their CCMD and potentially even based in their same time zone (or at least a time zone that would offer them real-time access during their work hours, which is currently not the case).

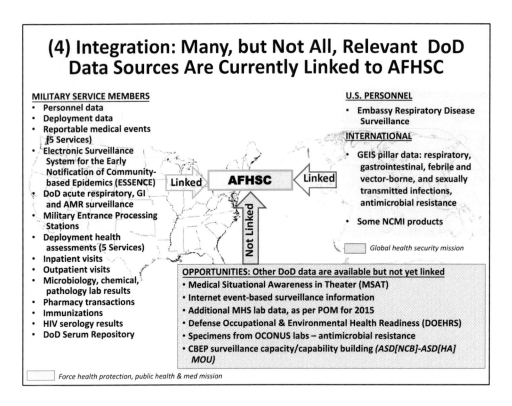

(4) Integration: Many, but Not All, Relevant DoD Data Sources Are Currently Linked to AFHSC

MILITARY SERVICE MEMBERS
- Personnel data
- Deployment data
- Reportable medical events (5 Services)
- Electronic Surveillance System for the Early Notification of Community-based Epidemics (ESSENCE)
- DoD acute respiratory, GI and AMR surveillance
- Military Entrance Processing Stations
- Deployment health assessments (5 Services)
- Inpatient visits
- Outpatient visits
- Microbiology, chemical, pathology lab results
- Pharmacy transactions
- Immunizations
- HIV serology results
- DoD Serum Repository

U.S. PERSONNEL
- Embassy Respiratory Disease Surveillance

INTERNATIONAL
- GEIS pillar data: respiratory, gastrointestinal, febrile and vector-borne, and sexually transmitted infections, antimicrobial resistance
- Some NCMI products

Global health security mission

Linked — **AFHSC** — Linked

Not Linked

OPPORTUNITIES: Other DoD data are available but not yet linked
- Medical Situational Awareness in Theater (MSAT)
- Internet event-based surveillance information
- Additional MHS lab data, as per POM for 2015
- Defense Occupational & Environmental Health Readiness (DOEHRS)
- Specimens from OCONUS labs – antimicrobial resistance
- CBEP surveillance capacity/capability building (ASD[NCB]-ASD[HA] MOU)

Force health protection, public health & med mission

The fourth dimension of biosurveillance system performance is integration (both internal within DoD and external), referring to the breadth of data available to a single DoD entity, such as AFHSC, and AFHSC's ability to combine relevant data streams across military Services and incorporate other types of data from DoD and non-DoD sources (e.g., CBEP-supported studies or biosurveillance capacity building, data from other federal agencies, inter-governmental organizations, non-government sources).

This figure depicts internal integration. AFHSC currently monitors and integrates data collected through DoD programs:

- AFHSC-supported biosurveillance in military and affiliated populations
- AFHSC collaboration to support biosurveillance in partner countries through GEIS.

AFHSC's DMSS incorporates a rich breadth of relevant data on military Service members. However, AFHSC has identified additional data that are available and should be linked. Their Program Objective Memorandum (POM) for 2015 identifies examples: medical situational awareness in theater, Internet event-based surveillance information, additional (unspecified) military health system laboratory information, and direct links to the DOEHRS.

Data and reports received through GEIS are also appropriately robust in terms of the syndromes monitored in the 63 countries worldwide. The 2012 Memorandum of Understanding (MOU) between ASD(NCB) and ASD(HA) that aims for closer collaboration between AFHSC and the CBEP programs will enhance exchange of relevant information of mutual benefit to both parties. In addition, AFHSC specifies in its POM for 2015 the desirability of more specimens from OCONUS labs for antimicrobial resistance testing—to complement the existing domestic system overseen by WRAIR.

Biosurveillance integration is both a policy and technical matter. The first hurdle is to identify and receive in one organization a wide range of relevant data. The second hurdle is the interoperability of information technology systems in which the data are collected, transmitted, and stored, i.e., efficient technical integration. Numerous DoD officials indicated more progress on the first hurdle than the second, with lack of interoperability of biosurveillance systems across the military Services the most prominent example.

More-efficient integration via knowledge management is a key need of CCMD surgeons, according to two public health professionals from one geographic CCMD. From their perspective in the field, the flow of information relevant to biosurveillance is inefficient and lacking a process. Multiple emails and groups will share the same piece of information, wasting considerable staff time. They would like to know "what is out there and how to get to it efficiently" and feel the need for more manpower to help them with data synthesis. Because there is no single biosurveillance program in DoD at this juncture, the community of practice relies on professional networks, emails, and phone calls. While this is working for now, a more formalized and institutionalized network and knowledge management system would create more efficiencies and connect the various stakeholders better. This might be an overlooked organizational opportunity for the DIB as it develops and evolves.

There is one important caveat to better integration of stakeholders across DoD. All of the actors recognize that a distinct distance must be maintained between the Intelligence Community and the health and bioweapons defense communities. All stakeholders recognize that the health and bioweapons defense operators will lose their credibility with key Ministry of Health officials in partner countries if they are perceived as linked to intelligence operations.

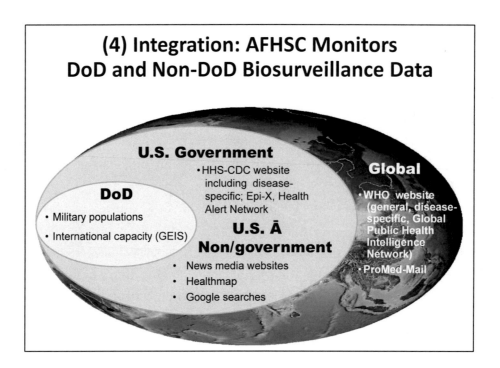

(4) Integration: AFHSC Monitors DoD and Non-DoD Biosurveillance Data

External integration extends beyond the organizational components and efforts of DoD itself. It takes into account—and often interfaces usefully with—programs and data from other federal departments and agencies. Because of the global nature of biosurveillance threats and DoD programming, DoD also takes into account relevant global biosurveillance information.

AFHSC monitors data collected by other federal agencies, non-government U.S. sources, and global sources, as shown in the figure above and in Table 3.1.

Table 3.1. Non-DoD Information Currently Monitored by AFHSC

Type of Source	Information Monitored
U.S. government	HHS/CDC: • Main website • Specific diseases/pathogens/syndromes (e.g., dengue, foodborne, influenza, fungal meningitis) • Global Disease Detection (GDD) Operations Center Daily Report (not open source) • Epi-X • Health Alert Network
U.S. non-government	General news media sites Program for Monitoring Emerging Diseases (ProMed-Mail) Healthmap Google searches
Global	WHO • Main website • Global Public Health Intelligence Network • Specific diseases/pathogens/syndromes • Global Polio Eradication Initiative

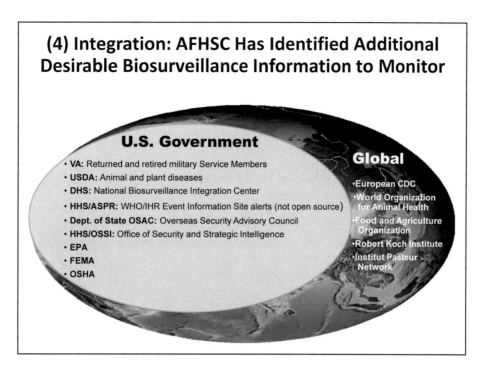

(4) Integration: AFHSC Has Identified Additional Desirable Biosurveillance Information to Monitor

U.S. Government

- **VA:** Returned and retired military Service Members
- **USDA:** Animal and plant diseases
- **DHS:** National Biosurveillance Integration Center
- **HHS/ASPR:** WHO/IHR Event Information Site alerts (not open source)
- **Dept. of State OSAC:** Overseas Security Advisory Council
- **HHS/OSSI:** Office of Security and Strategic Intelligence
- **EPA**
- **FEMA**
- **OSHA**

Global

- European CDC
- World Organization for Animal Health
- Food and Agriculture Organization
- Robert Koch Institute
- Institut Pasteur Network

AFHSC has identified additional information that it could monitor and integrate into its overall situational awareness, resources permitting (see figure above and Table 3.2). Some data come from organizations that monitor animal and plant diseases, which DoD does not; the study team added the Department of Veterans Affairs (VA) as another source of information pertaining to veterans, especially recent Service members, which may have implications for current Service members. Based on the prioritization of strategic-level missions, the highest priorities for these new links would be those most relevant to force health protection, followed by biological weapons defense and global health security.

Table 3.2. Potential Additional Information to Be Monitored by AFHSC

Source	Information to Be Monitored
U.S. government	• VA: Department of Veterans Affairs • U.S. Department of Agriculture: Animal and plant diseases • DHS: National Biosurveillance Integration Center • HHS/ASPR: alerts from the WHO/IHR Event Information Site, open only to Ministries of Health (not open source) • Department of State: Overseas Security Advisory Council • HHS: Office of Security and Strategic Intelligence • Environmental Protection Agency • DHS: Federal Emergency Management Agency • Office of Safety and Health Administration
Global	• European Center for Disease Prevention and Control • World Organization for Animal Health • Food and Agricultural Organization • Robert Koch Institute • Institut Pasteur network

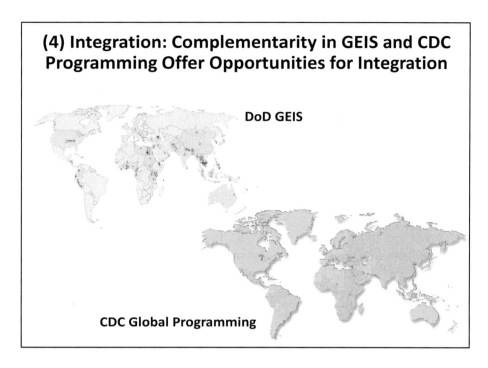

(4) Integration: Complementarity in GEIS and CDC Programming Offer Opportunities for Integration

DoD GEIS

CDC Global Programming

CDC also has extensive global programming relevant to biosurveillance and communicable disease prevention and control. The overlap and complementarity of GEIS and CDC global programming offer opportunities for coordination and integration of biosurveillance data and information between DoD and CDC.

For example, through overseas- and U.S.-based experts, CDC provides technical assistance related to biosurveillance, outbreak containment, public health system development, and training to foreign Ministries of Health. CDC also has long-standing and productive partnerships with multilateral health organizations, such as WHO.

CDC specifically addresses the following in its global programming:

- HIV/AIDS
- malaria
- neglected tropical diseases
- influenza
- polio
- immunizations
- emerging infectious diseases
- tuberculosis

- micronutrient malnutrition
- safe water
- refugee health
- maternal and child health
- occupational safety and health
- laboratory systems and services
- toxic substances and hazardous wastes

Assessment of Outputs

AFHSC Produced >1000 Recurrent Reports in FY2012

Report Type	# of reports	Total # products / year (including multiple versions)
Disease	15	243
Vaccines	4	40
Deployment	16	135
Mental health	13	148
Injuries	11	95
Special	15	347
TOTAL	**74**	**1,008**

AFHSC produces more than 1,000 recurrent reports each year, in addition to ad hoc reports and journal publications (65 articles published in AFHSC's *Medical Surveillance Monthly Report* and 60 additional papers published in peer-reviewed journals during fiscal year 2012). In fiscal year 2012, AFHSC produced 74 different health-related surveillance reports, some in multiple versions, as summarized in the table shown here and detailed in Appendix F. The study team compiled this list from different documents provided by and subsequently validated with AFHSC. Recurrent reports are produced at frequencies ranging from weekly to monthly, quarterly, semi-annually, and annually. AFHSC produces no routine near-real-time reports for situational awareness purposes.

Several reports are produced in different versions: 96 total versions of the 74 different reports, total of 1,008 distinct products in fiscal year 2012. Of these, 15 different reports and 243 individual products are specifically related to communicable diseases: five weekly reports (communicable diseases – two, influenza – three), three monthly reports (malaria – two, meningococcus – one), and seven annual reports (for different pathogens or diseases). Four additional reports (40 distinct products) related to adverse effects from vaccines: three monthly reports (smallpox and anthrax, adenovirus, other vaccines – one each), and one quarterly report on adenovirus vaccine safety; DoD is the main U.S. user of adenovirus vaccine. Other recurrent reports relate to deployment (16 reports, 135 products), mental health (13 reports, 148 products), injuries (11 reports, 95 products), and special reports (15 reports, 347 products).

The Study Team Developed Criteria to Assess Biosurveillance Outputs

Output Attributes	Criteria
(1) Relevance	• Relevance of diseases/conditions reported to the military • Actionable information • Clearly understood by decision makers • Presentation format that is acceptable to decision makers • Convenient dissemination mode (e.g., push/pull) • Includes characterization and/or forecasting of progression/impact
(2) Reach	• Number and appropriateness of audience(s) receiving outputs/reports
(3) Completeness	• Covers the entire (or enough of the) population and/or geographic area of responsibility of the consumer
(4) Timeliness	• Outputs are issued and received at frequencies commensurate with mission need
(5) Integration	• Whether DoD outputs draw from internal (other DoD) and/or external sources (e.g., CDC, FDA, WHO)

The study team developed attributes and criteria to assess DoD biosurveillance outputs:

- Relevance: Refers to information produced that is actionable, clearly understood by decision makers, presented in a format that is acceptable to the decision makers, disseminated in a convenient mode (whether pushed out actively or made available online to "pull" as needed; written, graphic, and/or oral briefing), and whether the information includes characterization of an event and/or forecasting of progression/impact.
- Reach: Refers to the number and appropriateness of audience(s) receiving biosurveillance outputs/reports.
- Completeness: Refers to whether the output covers the entire population and/or geographic area of interest (or at least sufficiently so) for the consumer.
- Timeliness: Refers to timing of outputs that are issued and received at frequencies commensurate with need. For example, daily if needs are near-real-time; weekly to monthly or quarterly for needs that are not as time sensitive.
- Integration: Refers to whether and the degree to which DoD outputs draw from internal (other DoD) and/or external sources (e.g., CDC, Food and Drug Administration [FDA], WHO).

The Team Assessed a List of AFHSC Outputs Using These Criteria

Output Attribute	Findings
Relevance	Wide range of reports of military relevance produced by AFHSC (and similarly relevant reports produced by NCMI)
Reach	• Web access for 1 of 8 weekly reports, 1 of 30 monthly reports, and 7 of 16 annual reports • Weekly communicable disease reports reach at least 25 recipients, but cannot judge the adequacy of these numbers
Completeness	(List of recurrent AFHSC reports does not provide sufficient evidence to assess this criterion)
Timeliness	• Daily: None • Weekly: 8/74 (11 percent) • Monthly: 30/74 (41 percent) • Quarterly: 12/74 (16 percent) • Semi-annual: 3/74 (4 percent) • Annual: 16/74 (22 percent)
Integration	(List of recurrent AFHSC reports does not provide sufficient evidence to assess this criterion)

This assessment is based mainly on examination of the list of recurrent reports produced by AFHSC, characterized by category, frequency, and number (Appendix F). It also includes general information about reporting by NCMI. CBEP programming produces entirely different types of outputs, i.e., not biosurveillance reports per se. Therefore, the findings reflect biosurveillance reporting from AFHSC and NCMI. Key findings are as follows:

- Relevance: AFHSC produces a range of reports relevant to military health and force health protection. These are related to disease (15 different reports), vaccines (4), deployment (16), mental health (13), injury (11), and "special" (15). In addition, NCMI produces reports based on daily scanning of 70–80 diseases of military interest across 165 countries. Thus, the AFHSC and NCMI reports appear to cover an appropriate range of health issues relevant to the military. Staff from one CCMD interviewed by the study team indicate that there is a great deal of relevant reporting, but they perceive that some of the information is not directed at the operational needs of the CCMD. Further, there is a significant amount of irrelevant (to the CCMD) information that they receive from across the stakeholder community. In sum, there appears to be a knowledge management issue, most likely due to the fact that the DoD biosurveillance enterprise is neither currently unified nor sufficiently integrated.
- Reach: The two weekly communicable disease reports produced by AFHSC reach 42 and 27 recipients, and the weekly influenza report reaches 108 recipients and is also available on the web (i.e., virtually unlimited reach). All of the annual disease reports, the one annual mental health report and one monthly injury report are also available on the web. According to AFHSC, several reports reach only one customer each.
- Completeness: The list of recurrent reports produced by AFHSC does not provide sufficient evidence for assessing this criterion. In general, however, reports reflecting health conditions in military Service members are more complete than reports from partner countries. NCMI characterizes its products as typically "early and incomplete;"

however, NCMI's timely assessments, albeit with incomplete data, play a vital role in situational awareness.

- Timeliness: AFHSC produces 74 different recurrent reports, some in multiple versions. Of the 74, eight (11 percent) are weekly; 30 (41 percent) are monthly; 12 (16 percent) are quarterly; 3 (4 percent) are semi-annual; and 16 (22 percent) are annual. AFHSC produces no daily reports. As noted earlier, NCMI produces assessments based on daily scans of numerous relevant diseases across most countries worldwide. Importantly, while not conveying an official view, the CCMD staff members with whom the study team spoke indicated that they are not receiving information in a sufficiently timely manner, and that they have trouble using the products offered to them from both NCMI and the AFHSC to influence decisions.
- Integration: The listing of AFHSC reports did not provide the evidence needed to assess the degree to which reports incorporate data from other DoD entities or external data monitored by AFHSC.

The Study Team Developed Criteria to Assess Inputs -- Biosurveillance Enterprise Enabling Functions

Enabling Functions	Criteria
(1) Doctrine and policy	• Congress or SECDEF has mandated/provided authority • Clear roles and responsibilities are adequately established across the biosurveillance enterprise • Organizational relationships are mandated
(2) Governance	• Governing body/bodies exist and have authorities required to assign and adjudicate roles and responsibilities
(3) Organizational Structures	• "Joint" where appropriate and beneficial
(4) People	• Staffing is authorized through manning document • Sufficient numbers • Appropriate qualifications
(5) Facilities	• Office and lab space and specimen storage are adequate
(6) Materiel	• Information technology systems and laboratories are adequate to fulfill mission
(7) Logistics	• Key systems are interoperable with relevant AFHSC system • Access to relevant classified data

Using the Joint Capabilities Integration Development framework known as DOTMLPF (doctrine, organization, training, materiel, leadership and education, personnel, facilities), the study team examined the enabling functions of the current biosurveillance enterprise:

- Doctrine and policy: First, the team examined what authorities underlie each of the primary lines of effort and stakeholders in the current enterprise. The team examined U.S. Code, national policy documents, and DoD Directives (DoDDs) and Instructions to determine what the DoD's missions, roles and responsibilities are for each organization and how those organizations are directed to relate to each other.
- Governance: Next, the team examined what governing or oversight bodies are mandated to be established for the current enterprise, and how those governing bodies are constructed.
- Organizational structures: The study team also examined whether there is an appropriate joint office of responsibility, and whether the organizations currently engaged have appropriate manning for their current mission as well as for an expansion of mission.
- Personnel: The team looked at where the availability of human resources within the biosurveillance enterprise might hinder further expansion—from the expert end of the scale to the lower end of expertise. Growing highly talented expertise takes time and money.
- Facilities, Materiel, Logistics: The team also looked at the ability of facilities, information systems, laboratories and other logistics systems to support the current biosurveillance enterprise as well as their ability to support an expansion.

(1) Doctrine/Policy: The First Specific Biosurveillance Guidance Was Issued in June 2013

- Deputy Secretary of Defense issued interim guidance for implementing the National Strategy for Biosurveillance on June 13, 2013
  - Calls for actions to "integrate, synchronize, and coordinate biosurveillance activities at the tactical, operational, and strategic levels and to enable sharing and receiving of biosurveillance information with external partners"
  - Calls for submission of a DoD Directive for biosurveillance within 12 months
- Because most of this study was carried out before the June 2013 guidance, RAND examined statutes and policies relative to existing functional areas

As previously noted, until the Deputy Secretary of Defense issued interim guidance on June 13, 2013, for implementation of the National Strategy for Biosurveillance, DoD had no explicit doctrine or policy that addressed biosurveillance, nor did it use the term "biosurveillance" in any directive documents. The June 2013 interim guidance specifically calls for actions to "integrate, synchronize, and coordinate biosurveillance activities at the tactical, operational, and strategic levels and to enable sharing and receiving of biosurveillance information with external partners" (OSD, 2013); it also calls for the submission of a DoDD for biosurveillance within 12 months. The memo places the DoD biosurveillance enterprise squarely within the context of the National Biosurveillance Strategy and begins to formalize the DoD biosurveillance enterprise.

Most of this study was carried out before the June 2013 guidance began to establish specific biosurveillance policy for DoD. Therefore, the study team examined policy and doctrine from each of the three lines of effort described previously: health surveillance, host-nation biosurveillance capacity/capability building, and medical intelligence.

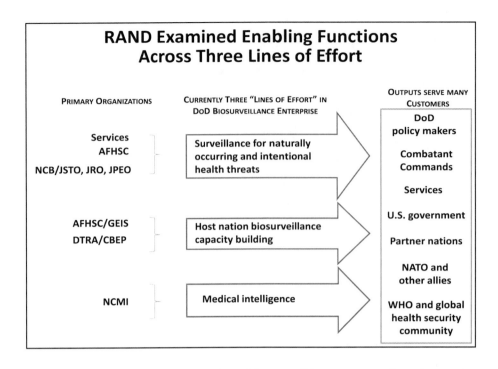

Referring back to the initial depiction of the biosurveillance enterprise, the study team examined the enabling functions that support each of the stakeholders in their primary lines of effort, using a DOTMLPF construct (Doctrine, Organization, Training, materiel, Leadership, Personnel, Facilities). The stakeholders are listed on the left side of each arrow.

(1)Doctrine/Policy: The Authorities for Current Lines of Effort Lack Clear Relational Directives

Lines of Effort	Health Surveillance	Host Nation Capacity/Capability Building	Medical Intelligence
Organizations / programs	AFHSC, ASD(NCB)	GEIS, CBEP	NCMI
U.S. Code or national policy authorities?	Yes – Title 10, Chapter 55 Force Health Protection; Title 50, Section 1522 Chem Bio Defense	Yes- Title 50 USC Chem/Bio Defense Program; NSTC-7 on Emerging Infectious Disease (authorizes GEIS)	Yes- Title 50 USC, Chapters 33 and 36, as well as PL 108-456 all on Intelligence Capacity of the U.S. government
Clear roles and responsibilities for functional area?	Yes	Yes	Yes
Relationships between stakeholders clearly delineated?	No—but recent ASD(HA)-ASD(NCB) MOU establishes relationship	No—but recent ASD (HA)-ASD(NCB) MOU establishes relationship	Yes

The study team examined authorities organized around the current functional lines of effort. Each of the major stakeholders reported that they feel they have sufficient lines of authority for their main efforts, and responsibilities within those three main lines are relatively well spelled out.

The primary issue surrounds the relationships between the entities, particularly between AFHSC and ASD(NCB). However, the ASD's for Health Affairs (HA) and ASD(NCB) signed a Memorandum of Understanding (MOU) in 2012 which establishes a framework (and has a corresponding operational plan) for a formal relationship between these two entities and the relevant programming under them. Connections between operational and intelligence agencies must be carefully managed.

```
┌─────────────────────────────────────────────────────────────┐
│                    (2) Governance:                          │
│               Multiple Mechanisms Exist                     │
│                                                             │
│  Formal                                                     │
│   • Health surveillance is governed by the Force Health     │
│     Integration Council under ASD(HA)                       │
│   • June 2013 interim guidance for implementation of the    │
│     National Strategy for Biosurveillance appoints          │
│     Biological Preparedness Group to coordinate tasks       │
│     specified in the guidance                               │
│                                                             │
│  Informal                                                   │
│   • ASD(HA) and ASD(NCB) meet regularly to discuss status   │
│     of MOU implementation                                   │
│   • Combatant Commands contribute to the consideration of   │
│     AFHSC/GEIS projects that will be funded in their area   │
│     of responsibility                                       │
│                                                             │
└─────────────────────────────────────────────────────────────┘
```

The second enabling function is governance. The study team found that while each line of effort has a specific set of working groups to help govern their activities, to date there is not one single authority to oversee the entire biosurveillance enterprise.

Formal governance mechanisms include the Force Health Protection Integration Council under the ASD(HA), which has governed health surveillance, and the Biological Preparedness Group, which the Deputy Secretary of Defense's interim guidance issued on June 13, 2013, appoints as the coordinator for implementation of the tasks specified in the guidance. That group is co-chaired by the Assistant Secretary of Defense for Health Affairs, the Assistant Secretary of Defense for Nuclear, Chemical, and Biological Defense, the Assistant Secretary of Defense for Global Strategic Affairs, the Assistant Secretary of Defense for Homeland Defense and Americas' Security Affairs, and the Under Secretary of Defense for Intelligence.

Informal governance includes regular meetings of the ASD(HA) and the ASD(NCB) to discuss the status of implementation of their MOU and the contributions of the CCMDs to consideration of AFHSC/GEIS projects that will be funded in their respective areas of responsibility.

- The Military Health System is currently undergoing a re-structuring to create the Defense Health Agency, under the ASD(HA) chain of command

- AFHSC is the center of expertise within DoD for health surveillance functions

- AFHSC's Division of Integrated Biosurveillance is the hub for a more efficient and integrated DoD biosurveillance enterprise

The third enabling function is organization. At the same time that a DoDD is being developed to define formal policy for the biosurveillance enterprise, the Military Health System (MHS) is undergoing restructuring that will result in the creation of the DHA.

Within DoD, AFHSC has the greatest concentration of health surveillance expertise and experience and also the most biosurveillance-relevant systems and outputs. The MOU between the ASD(NCB) and the ASD(HA) also recognizes the role of AFHSC in the important collaboration between the programs under their respective chains of command.

One of three possible courses of action under the formalization of both the DHA and the DoD biosurveillance enterprise is to place AFHSC directly under that agency and designate it as the center of the DoD biosurveillance enterprise. In 2012 AFHSC created the DIB to serve as the 'belly button' for a reorganized and more efficient DoD biosurveillance enterprise, including expansion. Documentation from the DIB indicates three functional areas:

- alert and response operations
- communications, coordination, and engagement
- innovation and evaluation.

All of these factors suggest that AFHSC is a logical organization to serve as the center for the evolving DoD biosurveillance enterprise.

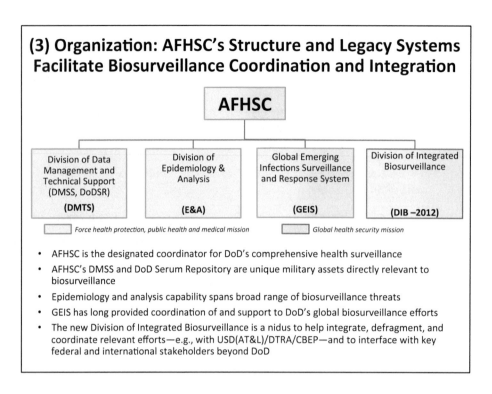

(3) Organization: AFHSC's Structure and Legacy Systems Facilitate Biosurveillance Coordination and Integration

- AFHSC is the designated coordinator for DoD's comprehensive health surveillance
- AFHSC's DMSS and DoD Serum Repository are unique military assets directly relevant to biosurveillance
- Epidemiology and analysis capability spans broad range of biosurveillance threats
- GEIS has long provided coordination of and support to DoD's global biosurveillance efforts
- The new Division of Integrated Biosurveillance is a nidus to help integrate, defragment, and coordinate relevant efforts—e.g., with USD(AT&L)/DTRA/CBEP—and to interface with key federal and international stakeholders beyond DoD

AFHSC's organizational structure, designated responsibilities to date, and legacy systems make it well-suited to coordinate and integrate DoD biosurveillance.

Especially important legacy systems include the Defense Medical Surveillance System and the DoD Serum Repository for military populations, both managed by the Division of Data Management and Technical Support. These support the strategic force health protection mission.

Epidemiologic analysis, managed by AFHSC's Division of Epidemiology and Analysis, is a core function of biosurveillance and military health surveillance.

GEIS is a key DoD program for global biosurveillance; GEIS supports both force health protection and global health security missions.

The new (since 2012) AFHSC DIB serves as a hub for absorbing the current and future requirements of coordinating and integrating biosurveillance across DoD. It also monitors the data of and interfaces with key federal and international stakeholders beyond DoD.

> **(4) Personnel:**
> **Human Capital Is the Primary Constraint**
>
> - AFHSC does not have the manpower to support expansion of its role
>   - It currently does not have a Manning Document consistent with present or future funding or mission
>   - Implementation of the MOU with the ASD(NCB) is constrained by AFHSC's manpower shortage
> - The expertise required for expansion of the DoD biosurveillance enterprise is quite high (e.g., epidemiologists and other scientists with military backgrounds) and will most likely require significant attention as DoD formalizes biosurveillance plans
> - The overseas lab capacity is also constrained by personnel ceilings of the respective embassies. AFHSC reports that the labs have significant potential but are constrained by the number of personnel able to work at the labs

The fourth enabling function is personnel. According to AFHSC staff and the office of the ASD(NCB), AFHSC has a critical manpower shortage to complete its current mission, which officially is force health protection, and for the global health security mission it also addresses. The AFHSC conducted a manpower survey in February 2012 that found that the organization requires 134 personnel to perform its role as the primary military health surveillance organization, although the organization is currently only authorized 42 staff (with 50 required) on the current Table of Distribution and Allowances and is currently functioning with 78 employees. The RAND team did not validate or verify the findings of the manpower survey, but it stands to reason that implementing the requirements and expanded mission of the ASD(NCB)-ASD(HA) MOU, the AFHSC will need more personnel.

Furthermore, tied to the development of the DIB, AFHSC has identified a critical need for additional manpower and expertise if its role in biosurveillance is to expand, i.e., in the interest of a more efficient and integrated DoD biosurveillance enterprise. Given its defined role as the DoD hub for biosurveillance integration, the DIB is the appropriate organization to take on the central coordination role as the DoD biosurveillance enterprise is formalized. However, the DIB presently has only seven personnel, and therefore is only able to handle a limited amount of either bureaucratic or biosurveillance work. The CCMD staff interviewed by the study team indicated a need for a dedicated staff person responsible for their area of operations who would be available during the same working hours as the CCMD; they further opined that manpower was the key limiter of current biosurveillance efforts.

Expansion of the DIB into a robust organization able to take on an expanded role is a critical need for the success of the entire enterprise. However, DIB expansion is uncertain under the current circumstances. Furthermore, AFHSC has no Manning Document, and therefore has a piecemeal system for filling personnel requirements. Creation of the DHA could increase manning and funding opportunities for the AFHSC by leveraging savings elsewhere in the public health systems of the Services. This will only become a more critical issue to the success of the biosurveillance enterprise as its mission-relevant activities become more robust and AFHSC takes on presumably larger coordination and data integration roles. DoD policy makers will have to consider expansion of AFHSC (including the DIB) in conjunction with the resource-constrained environment; risks to other missions; and payoffs for force health protection, biological weapons defense, and global health security missions. Also at issue is the timing of the reorganization of the MHS, which is unclear. Further, should manpower and resources become available to leverage into an increased capacity in the DIB, it will still be necessary for DoD policy makers to set and operationalize this as a priority, to support the entire biosurveillance enterprise.

Related to this manpower shortage, both AFHSC and ASD(NCB) staff reported that lack of critical manpower within AFHSC constrains implementation of the ASD(HA)-ASD(NCB) MOU. Furthermore, the expertise needed at the strategic level of organization is quite high, and not easily found. Finally, AFHSC reports that manpower at the overseas labs is also constrained by agreements with each embassy, a restriction that has operational effects working against global health security.

The fifth, sixth, and seventh enabling functions are facilities, materiel, and logistics. AFHSC is currently located in a commercial office park in central Maryland, just north of the District of Columbia, along with the DoD Serum Repository. Presently, the AFHSC does not have a classified computing capability nor does it currently have a secure facility for classified terminals. AFHSC told the study team that it plans to construct a small Secure Internet Protocol Router Network (SIPRnet) terminal room where staff can check their secure email, but such a terminal will only support classified communications with other DoD entities using primarily SIPRnet. Finally, the AFHSC is considering its need for a more real-time biohazard monitoring and alert capability, which might necessitate a specific facility. Should the AFHSC expand its staffing, the AFHSC leadership has indicated that they would need expanded space to support the increased staffing level. While the RAND team did not verify this, it only makes sense that facilities requirements would be tailored to the objectives of the organization.

Also, as previously discussed, data and information flows can serve to integrate organizations, and are critical to a fully enabled biosurveillance enterprise. There appears to be no central knowledge management system, although a few systems are in development by ASD(NCB), considering AFHSC a primary consumer of the developed product. Currently, however, the various stakeholders have a significant amount of inefficiency in their information and data collection and use. This "noise" might be reduced if the various stakeholders had a specific knowledge management system (which could be based on many of the DoD technical solutions already developed) with business rules.

Key Findings

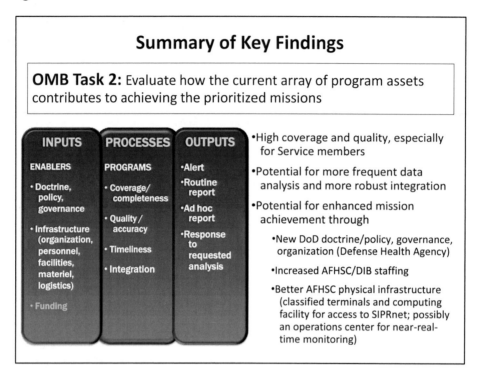

Assessment of the performance of DoD biosurveillance systems and processes indicates that

- DoD health surveillance population and data coverage for military Service members are comprehensive; they support DoD's force health protection mission.
- DoD biosurveillance population and data coverage internationally cover syndromes and pathogens of relevance to partner countries and DoD; they support both the force health protection and global health security missions of DoD, and also the broader U.S. government and global health security communities.
- The quality of DoD biosurveillance is higher than typical public health surveillance because of the availability of denominator data, standardized case definitions, and the high quality and high degree of testing performed by DoD laboratories; however, since biosurveillance data are not fully validated, quality may not be as consistently high as expected.
- AFHSC undertakes very little routine near-real-time data analysis and reporting for situational awareness purposes. More frequent analyses and some additional data linkages could further enhance the value of DoD biosurveillance, especially for current situational awareness. The final operating capability for AFHSC's DIB includes more staff and plans for daily analyses and situational reports if resources become available.

The most important opportunities for improvement in system performance are summarized in Table 3.3.

Table 3.3. Opportunities to Improve DoD Biosurveillance System Performance

System Attributes	Opportunities
Coverage/Completeness	• Harnessing the assessments from NCMI, and relevant results from CBEP-supported studies
Quality/Accuracy	• Validation of biosurveillance data • Approaches to encourage full and open reporting (e.g., of mental illness or other perceived stigmatizing conditions) on deployment health assessments
Timeliness	• More near-real-time data transmission and analysis of data on Service members if/as warranted, in support of situational awareness and the force health protection mission • Approaches to increase frequency of global biosurveillance data analysis by GEIS partners (e.g., in countries, at GEIS headquarters)
Integration	• Additional data linkages for biosurveillance in military Service members (as identified by AFHSC) • Increased range of non-DoD information monitored by DoD (AFHSC has identified relevant desired information)

The current DoD biosurveillance enterprise exists across myriad functional areas in DoD, and as of the date of this report there is no unifying doctrine or policy, nor any formalized governance structure or process. The interim guidance issued by the Deputy Secretary of Defense on June 13, 2013 for implementation of the National Strategy for Biosurveillance is a good start toward unifying the various actors, de-conflicting roles and responsibilities, and structuring oversight organizations and processes. Meanwhile, the department has formed a Biological Preparedness Group that is examining ways to implement the National Strategy for Biosurveillance, and each functional area (intelligence, health, and bioweapons defense) has a stake in the working group. The June 2013 interim guidance appointed this group to coordinate the tasks specified in the guidance.

The MOU between the ASD(HA) and ASD(NCB) recognizes AFHSC as the center for the emerging biosurveillance capability. AFHSC has established the DIB to oversee integration of biosurveillance efforts across DoD. The limiting enabler for the AFHSC, and therefore for the entire enterprise, is manpower. Not only is the DIB understaffed for its aspirational role in the biosurveillance enterprise, but it appears to be understaffed for its current role within the AFHSC—including its responsibilities under the ASD(HA)-ASD(NCB) MOU—having only seven personnel. In addition to the criticality of the manpower shortage within the AFHSC is the need for appropriately qualified analysts. The level of expertise required is somewhat extraordinary in that the personnel must have technical health and epidemiological expertise as well as extensive understanding of the DoD enterprise and even expertise in the broader range of U.S. government and international organizations and programming related to global health security.

Not only does the AFHSC require an investment in manpower, it currently lacks classified terminals and a classified facility to better communicate with other surveillance partners and customers. Ready access to DoD's classified data systems would enable AFHSC to capture a more robust range of relevant data. Also, AFHSC clearly has a requirement to improve its near- real-time monitoring of threats and emerging biological events, and to this end it is studying the feasibility of establishing an alert and response capability. This might be accomplished in many ways, but the requirement to improve monitoring and response times is clear. A summary of opportunities related to the enablers of DoD's biosurveillance is presented in Table 3.4.

Table 3.4. Summary of Opportunities Related to Biosurveillance System Enablers

Enabling Functions	Opportunities
Doctrine and policy	June 2013 interim guidance begins to establish DoD doctrine specifically for biosurveillance: Adopts definition used in National Strategy for Biosurveillance (implications are yet unclear regarding expansion beyond purely human health); forthcoming DoDD will define key terms and designate roles and responsibilities
Governance	Establish governance for biosurveillance that ensures efficiency, compliance, and integration
Organization	Establish an oversight body with the authority to adjudicate roles and responsibilities overlaps, resource constraints and other issues that normally arise in a cross-functional endeavor
People	Ensure adequate manning resources for DoD biosurveillance, most critically, staffing for AFHSC
Facilities	Ensure sufficient classified computing space and facilities to support an expansion of the AFHSC capability for near real-time monitoring and alert of emerging threats, including data transmitted through DoD's classified systems
Materiel	Establish on-site access by AFHSC to classified data feeds relevant to biosurveillance
Logistics	Address information technology issues, including interoperability, to enhance timeliness and efficiency of data collection, transmission, and integration. A knowledge management role should be designated, business rules developed, and the effort should be based on an existing technological solution already available within DoD.

4. OMB Task 3—Funding

OMB Task 3: Assess whether the current funding system is appropriate and how it can be improved to ensure stable funding

Findings:

- Explicit authority, suitable structural and functional organization, and a governance mechanism that enables visibility and coordination of funding streams across the DoD biosurveillance enterprise can enhance its efficiency and effectiveness.
- ASD(NCB) staff expressed that they are resourced to sustain their current missions.
- NCMI expects significant cuts in the next fiscal year.
- AFSHC is resourced to sustain current operations but has requested additional funding to fully implement its responsibilities under the ASD(HA)-ASD(NCB) MOU. With additional responsibilities for coordinating the entire DoD biosurveillance enterprise, it is only natural that it would need concomitant resourcing.

Methods for OMB Task 3: Funding

OMB Task 3: Assess whether the current funding system is appropriate and how it can be improved to ensure stable funding.

- Develop and apply criteria to assess appropriateness and stability of DoD biosurveillance funding system
- Examine relevant program documentation
  - AFHSC 2014 unfunded request, POM submission, and TMA MEDCOM Base Funding documentation
  - DTRA/CBEP budget history
  - FY 2014 NCB budget, separating out Joint Biodefense Program (Medical) and Contamination Avoidance Program expenditures, which were generally most relevant to the biosurveillance enterprise
- Discuss perceived funding stability with the three main actors
- Did NOT conduct rigorous budget analysis to identify effectiveness, redundancies or possible efficiencies across funding streams

---

To complete the funding assessment called for in OMB Task 3, the study team first developed criteria for assessing the appropriateness and stability of the DoD biosurveillance funding system. This is explained later in this section.

Next, the team examined budget documents provided by AFHSC along with information provided by NCMI and the office of the ASD(NCB). An examination of the DoD budget for the past three years also provided details for understanding the funding streams and systems.

73

Specifically, the team examined the AFHSC budget request documents provided by the AFHSC and the July 15, 2013, Tricare Management Activity (TMA) U.S. Army Medical Command (MEDCOM) Base Funding document, as well as the fiscal year 2014 budget for the Chemical and Biological Defense Program, which is publicly available on the DoD Comptroller's webpage. The team also examined documentation on the Chemical and Biological Defense Program Research Development Test and Evaluation budget. It was not feasible to separate out the purely biosurveillance-relevant budget, though this report includes summary figures in a table later in this section. Further, the study team examined budget documentation on the CBEP.

The study team also discussed budget streams with the AFHSC and their parent organization, the office of the DASD(FHP&R), NCMI, the office of the ASD(NCB), and the CBEP to understand their perception of their budget environment.

Finally, it is important to note that the study team did not conduct a budget analysis to look for efficiencies or to examine whether the streams that fund the DoD biosurveillance enterprise are effectively supporting programs and producing the desired outcomes.

Attributes	Criteria
The Study Team Developed Criteria to Assess the Appropriateness and Stability of Funding Systems	
Appropriateness: Ability to allocate resources efficiently, effectively across the enterprise	• Oversight mechanism • Aligned to support common objectives identified across the enterprise • Ability to shift resources across functional areas according to emerging needs
Stability	• Recent budget history (budget stability over past three years) • Perceived stability of near-term future budgets

OMB Task 3 asks whether the current funding system is appropriate and how it can be improved to ensure stable funding.

An appropriate funding system will relate expenditures to achievement of objectives (Schick, 1996). Therefore the attributes of an appropriate biosurveillance enterprise funding system are the ability to allocate resources efficiently and effectively across the entire biosurveillance enterprise. As Allen Schick, the preeminent budget scholar, wrote, "Every budget system, even rudimentary ones, comprises planning, management and control processes" (Schick, 1996).

Drawing from Schick, the study team established the following criteria for examining the funding system of the DoD biosurveillance enterprise:

- The enterprise funding system should have an oversight mechanism to plan, manage and control the system.
- The enterprise funding system should be aligned to support common objectives of the enterprise.
- The funding system should be able to shift funds across various programs in order to meet emergent needs.

Finally, the study team determined that the stability of the funding system would be characterized by the past three years of the program's budget history, combined with perceptions of key stakeholders regarding whether future budgets will be reflective of those recent past budgets. The leadership perspective is particularly important because DoD's budgets are undergoing significant change and the past three years are not necessarily reflective of the next year, not to mention the next three years. Nonetheless, the budget history of the organizations involved in the biosurveillance enterprise can demonstrate trends from which we might infer prioritization.

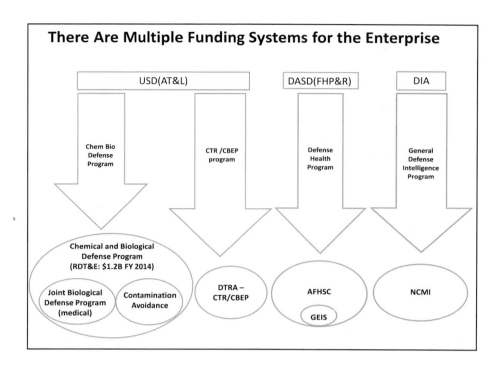

There Are Multiple Funding Systems for the Enterprise

DoD has a considerable investment in the biosurveillance enterprise. There are multiple funding systems that support the current DoD biosurveillance enterprise, yet no overarching mechanism with the authority to coordinate allocation of funds across the entire enterprise in a way to meet overarching goals, nor to meet emerging needs. The funding systems that support each of the contributing organizations function well within those particular domains; however, an overall funding system is absent.

There are four funding systems that make up the current 'system' for the enterprise. The four primary funding systems along with the organization responsible for that funding line are depicted in the figure above, and, within each of those funding systems, there are respective authorities that can manage the funds according to the priorities and requirements of each system. Through its examination of budget lines, the study team could certainly see how various efforts are supportive of the entire enterprise and mission accomplishment, as described below. Finally, the funding streams for the stakeholders appear to be relatively steady, with the exception of the significant cuts being predicted for NCMI. Stakeholders reported that they have sufficient funds with which to support their current responsibilities; however, the office of the ASD(NCB) and AFHSC point to critical shortages in the AFHSC. In particular, the office of the ASD(NCB) has pointed to critical shortfalls in the ability of the AFHSC to implement its additional responsibilities under the ASD(HA)-ASD(NCB) MOU.

AFHSC receives Defense Health Program funds from the DASD(FHP&R) to support both its epidemiological activities as well as the global health activities of GEIS. As an example of how the funding system of the entire enterprise is not able to respond to emerging needs, the AFHSC has developed a request for a $7 million increase in annual funding to increase its capabilities to support the full implementation of the MOU with the ASD(NCB). This funding would support the addition of 15 full-time equivalent employees, allow the AFHSC to integrate classified data and reporting into its operations, and would support the development of a real-time monitoring and alert capability and facility. These suggested budget increases do not enhance the AFHSC's ability to expand the portfolio of pathogens that it monitors, and the AFHSC has proposed an additional seven unfunded requirements for a total of $18.35 million per year for five years, beginning in fiscal year 2015. The study team did not validate or verify the analysis that AFHSC has provided. Nonetheless, the office of the ASD(NCB) has suggested that the ability to fully formalize the biosurveillance enterprise and fully implement the ASD(NCB)-ASD(HA) MOU is hindered by critical resource shortfalls in AFHSC.

NCMI receives its funding through the General Defense Intelligence Program via the DIA. The exact budget is classified.

The CBEP, which is in the DTRA portfolio, receives funds through the CTR program (DTRA, 2013). DTRA's funding for CTR/CBEP over the past three years has continued to grow, as shown in Table 4.1, although this program contributes to the global health security mission set, which is lower in priority than force health protection.

The Joint Biological Defense Program (medical) is a separate line item in the DoD budget under the overarching Nuclear, Chemical, and Biological Defense Program, and includes (1) the Advanced Anticonvulsant System, which consists of development of a new anti-convulsant agent; 2) the Next Generation Diagnostic System (NGDS), which is a medical test and diagnostic system that will be fielded to all Services and will identify biological warfare agents and pathogens of operational concern (NDGS will be discussed below); (3) DoD Biological Vaccines procurement; (4) a critical reagents program; and (5) biosurveillance requirements to address medical and physical chemical, biological, radiological, and nuclear mission needs for the Joint Biosurveillance Common Framework, which will provide a single enterprise environment to support collaboration, data sharing, and coordination between multiple biosurveillance stakeholders (DoD, 2013b).

The NGDS (a part of the Joint Biological Defense Program) is of particular interest. In fiscal year 2013, the total cost for NGDS was $26.93 million; the fiscal year 2014 budget is $3.31 million. The next NGDS increment is intended to replace a legacy system—the Joint Biological Agent Identification and Diagnostic System (JBAIDS)—beginning in fiscal year 2017. The NGDS Increment 1 Service Laboratory Component is intended to provide high throughput threat identification, characterization, and diagnostics to CONUS and OCONUS laboratories. The subsequent increment will provide advanced diagnostics for biological pathogens and toxins, diagnostics for chemical and radiological exposures, and provide capabilities to low echelons of care. This program, therefore, demonstrates the nexus between the Services and the AFHSC and the ASD(NCB)'s Biological Weapons Defense Program, although it is not clear whether the funding oversight is sufficient to ensure that this planned capability can be implemented by the labs, and in particular the OCONUS labs (DoD, 2013b).

Another example of the support the biological defense program provides to biosurveillance enterprise is the Joint USFK (U.S. Forces, Korea) Portal and Integrated Threat Recognition (JUPITR) technological demonstration, which also is part of the Joint Biological Defense Program (medical). The JUPITR system, being developed for U.S. Pacific Command (USPACOM), will provide a platform to communicate, share data, and collaborate, from laboratory to operational use on countermeasures and techniques for countering biological threats. The Biosurveillance Portal, which is supported by the fiscal year 2014 budget, is the first installment of this system. The study team examined DoD documents that explore the requirements of the CCMDs for more precise biosurveillance informatics, yet these do not mention this platform as a solution. Therefore it is unclear whether the investment will be fully realized across the department to its fullest (DoD, 2013b).

The Contamination Avoidance procurement budget line item encompasses programs involved in the early detection, warning, and reporting and reconnaissance of biological and chemical threats. It is impossible to separate the chemical systems from the biological since the programs generally address both simultaneously, with the exception of the "Joint Chemical Agent Detector," which is not included in the overall Contamination Avoidance line item totals displayed in the figure above. Apart from this one exclusion, the rest of this line item includes (1) the Joint Biological Point Detection System, which consists of a trigger, sampler, detector, and identification technologies to detect and identify biological agents in real time; (2) the Non-Traditional Agent Detection Program to evaluate and test developmental technologies that enhance detection systems' capabilities to detect non-traditional agents; (3) the Joint Warning and Reporting Network, which provides an automated nuclear, chemical, and biological detection and warning process in a battlespace; (4) the Software Support Activity, which provides enterprise-wide services and coordination for interoperability; (5) the Joint Nuclear, Biological, and Chemical Reconnaissance Systems that support the Stryker Nuclear, Biological, and Chemical platform; and (6) the Chemical Biological Radiological and Nuclear Dismounted Reconnaissance Systems to detect, identify, sample, and mark nuclear, biological, and chemical hazards (DoD, 2013b).

The overall funding for the Chemical and Biological Defense Program Research, Development, Test, and Evaluation Expenditures is $1.2 billion, and a significant portion of that budget appears applicable to the DoD biosurveillance enterprise. However, the study team was not able to assess what amounts of the funds were specifically applicable and explicitly excluded R&D as out of scope for this report.

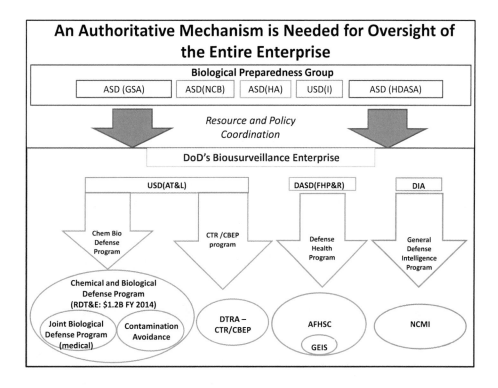

An Authoritative Mechanism is Needed for Oversight of the Entire Enterprise

Biological Preparedness Group

| ASD (GSA) | ASD(NCB) | ASD(HA) | USD(I) | ASD (HDASA) |

Resource and Policy Coordination

DoD's Biousurveillance Enterprise

USD(AT&L) — DASD(FHP&R) — DIA

Chem Bio Defense Program — CTR /CBEP program — Defense Health Program — General Defense Intelligence Program

Chemical and Biological Defense Program (RDT&E: $1.2B FY 2014)

Joint Biological Defense Program (medical) — Contamination Avoidance — DTRA – CTR/CBEP — AFHSC — NCMI

GEIS

On June 27, 2013, the White House issued the "Fiscal Year 2015 Budget Guidance for Countering Biological Threats Resource Priorities" and associated Global Health Security second-term agenda, which were developed by the National Security Staff in coordination with the OMB (White House, 2013). The purpose of the document is to help ensure that appropriate interagency resources are being allocated to priority global health security objectives, and it calls upon DoD (and other governmental agencies and departments) to identify which programs, projects, and activities align to the priorities. The fiscal year 2015 priorities outlined in the document are eight objectives under three main aims: (1) prevent avoidable epidemic, (2) detect threats early, and (3) respond rapidly and effectively to biological threats of international concern. This document highlights the criticality of an integrated biosurveillance effort, not only in DoD but across the federal government.

Within DoD, the funding streams for all organizations currently engaged in the biosurveillance enterprise are vulnerable to DoD budget cutbacks. As already discussed, NCMI is expecting significant cuts in fiscal year 2014. Because AFHSC receives its funding through the Defense Health Program, the priorities of that program provide an understanding of funding stability. The Defense Health Program documentation for fiscal year 2014 is silent on the matter of biosurveillance. This is not surprising given that biosurveillance is not a formal DoD effort and health surveillance is a supporting function of the overall public health endeavor—a line item in the Defense Health Program budget (DoD, 2013c).

Furthermore, although the MOU between the ASD(NCB) and the ASD(HA) expanded the AFHSC's role with respect to the overall enterprise, it is unclear whether the AFHSC will receive increased funding for its expanded responsibilities. The AFHSC leadership has expressed that its funding has been relatively stable in recent years, but current levels are insufficient for the additional responsibilities reflected in the MOU. The fiscal year 2014 Defense Health Program budget shows a $3 million planned increase, but it is not certain that this will be sustained in future years. The MHS is undergoing a reorganization into the Defense Health Agency, as previously described, which will reconfigure the public health functions currently resident in the Services. This reorganization may result in savings in resources and personnel that could then be shifted to the AFHSC. However, the timing of the changes and the willingness of the MHS leadership to prioritize biosurveillance is unclear, and savings realized by the reorganization could be shifted elsewhere. In contrast, the ASD(NCB) Defense Program budget documentation points to the National Strategy for Biosurveillance, and justifies the Joint Biological Defense Program budget, citing how expenditures in its portfolio map to the four capabilities of the strategy.

While appropriations generally come with restrictive rules about how funds may be spent, there might be avoidable redundancies and efficiencies to be found among the existing DoD funding systems and across federal agencies. Absent an authoritative DoD oversight mechanism, the parochial interests of each DoD organization in its separate funding system will continue to promote disjunctures between biosurveillance priorities and spending. Furthermore, multiple hierarchies within each funding stream also create inefficiencies as taxes and delays are created at each level of bureaucracy. An oversight organization with responsibility to match priorities and budgets within DoD and with the ability to find ways to leverage each resource stream for the benefit of the overall biosurveillance enterprise will be critical for its full and effective functioning. In particular, a central oversight authority must pay heed to the role and requirements of the AFHSC as the central operational coordinator for the nascent enterprise. Moreover, the DoD biosurveillance enterprise will require an authoritative mechanism for integrating DoD efforts and priorities with those of the rest of the government and to align efforts and spending with the greater U.S. government effort.

One possibility might be the existing Biological Preparedness Group, which the newly signed interim guidance on biosurveillance issued on June 13, 2013 by the Deputy Secretary of Defense appoints to oversee and coordinate implementation of the tasks in the guidance (OSD, 2013). This group is co-chaired by the ASD(HA), the ASD(NCB), the Assistant Secretary of Defense for Global Strategic Affairs, the Assistant Secretary of Defense for Homeland Defense and Americas' Security Affairs, and the Under Secretary of Defense for Intelligence. If this group is to continue serving in such a role, it would need a charter and process to provide oversight on DoD resourcing, and to also coordinate externally with the other federal agencies and departments involved in biosurveillance. The DoDD to be developed by June 2014 could specify such a role, for example.

Table 4.1 depicts budgets for fiscal years 2012–2014 for the funding systems described above. Although the funding context for the next several fiscal years is completely different than the previous three years, the table below illustrates the investment and commitment that DoD has already made to the biosurveillance enterprise.

Table 4.1. Budget History for Key DoD Biosurveillance-Related Programs, Fiscal Years 2012–2014

Program	Funding (in $ millions)*		
	2012	**2013**	**2014**
AFHSC	67.76 (AFHSC, 2013b)	69.23 (AFHSC, 2013b)	71.38 (AFHSC, 2013b)
DTRA/CBEP	229.47 (DTRA, 2013)	241.01 (estimated) (DTRA, 2013)	306.33 (estimated) (DTRA, 2013)
Chemical and Biological Defense Program Biosurveillance Investments**	155.73 (DoD, 2013a)	241.17 (DoD, 2013a)	249.02 (DoD, 2013a)

* All figures are pre-sequester.
** Figures from fiscal year 2014 Chemical and Biological Defense Program budget exhibits (diagnostics, environmental detection, and information technologies) that contribute to biosurveillance.

Key Findings

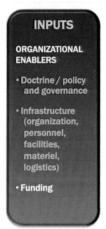

Summary of Key Findings

OMB Task 3: Assess whether the current funding system is appropriate and how it can be improved to ensure stable funding

INPUTS

ORGANIZATIONAL ENABLERS

- Doctrine / policy and governance
- Infrastructure (organization, personnel, facilities, materiel, logistics)
- Funding

- Explicit authority, suitable structural and functional organization, and a governance mechanism that enables visibility and coordination of funding streams across the DoD biosurveillance enterprise can enhance its efficiency and effectiveness
- ASD(NCB) staff expressed that they are resourced to sustain their current missions
- NCMI expects significant cuts in the next fiscal year
- AFSHC is resourced to sustain current operations but has requested additional funding to fully implement its responsibilities under the ASD(HA)-ASD(NCB) MOU. With additional responsibilities for coordinating the entire DoD biosurveillance enterprise, it is only natural that it would need concomitant resourcing

DoD has a considerable investment in the biosurveillance enterprise. The funding systems that support each of the contributing organizations function well within those particular domains. However, because there is no authoritative oversight mechanism for a biosurveillance enterprise at the time of this report, there is no coordination for allocation of funds across the entire enterprise in a way to meet overarching goals, nor to meet emerging needs. Furthermore, although biosurveillance and global health security are clearly White House priorities, as reflected in the guidance it issued for fiscal year 2015 budget priorities and alignment of relevant federal programs with these priorities, DoD currently has no ability to respond in a unified manner. Any oversight mechanism must have the ability to not only engage internally to DoD, but also to engage with the rest of the government.

Regarding stability, the AFHSC and the office of the ASD(NCB) have indicated that they expect relatively stable funding going forward in spite of the vulnerabilities and variations provided by the current cutbacks. The perception of the leadership within the AFHSC is that although they are resourced to sustain current operations, additional responsibilities associated with the ASD(HA)-ASD(NCB) MOU and meeting priorities and objectives of the National Strategy for Biosurveillance and the June 2013 White House guidance for fiscal year 2015 budget planning will require a concomitant expansion of resources. NCMI is expecting significant cuts, and the CBEP is experiencing increases in funding although it does not contribute as directly to the highest-priority mission of force health protection.

While there may still be funding shortages, it is not inconceivable that agencies could share resources to advance common objectives. The entire biosurveillance enterprise would likely benefit from an oversight organization, perhaps the existing Biological Preparedness Group, which the Deputy Secretary of Defense designated in his June 2013 interim guidance to oversee and coordinate tasks specified in the guidance. A more permanent and authoritative oversight and resource control role for this, or another appropriately constituted group, would help the entire enterprise by determining the feasibility and appropriateness of resource sharing, examining redundancies, and routinely reviewing and synchronizing the efforts of the stakeholders within the resource realities of DoD. Furthermore, such a body would need to have the authority to coordinate with other U.S. government agencies and departments working on biosurveillance. These will be important elements to address in the DoDD to be developed by June 2014.

5. Conclusions

Limitations

The Study Team Recognizes Important Limitations In This Report

- These results are limited by the relatively short time frame of the study during FY 2013

- The study team was not able to speak to some key stakeholders—such as more staff from the Combatant Commands, OSD (Policy), or in depth with more staff of the ASD(HA) and ASD(NCB)—to gain their perspectives as the consumers and budget holders of the biosurveillance enterprise, including their perspectives on the performance of biosurveillance

- The team may have missed or mischaracterized relevant programs or systems because there was no existing consolidated documentation of all of the information systems, data sources, data collection frequencies, and outputs that comprise the current biosurveillance effort

This report reflects facts and insights gleaned by the RAND team mainly during May–June 2013. The results may be limited by the relatively short time frame of the study.

The study team was able to speak with some key stakeholders from the CCMDs, ASD(HA), ASD(NCB), and NCMI, but might have benefitted from opportunities to speak with more of them and with staff from Under Secretary of Defense for Policy to gain their perspectives as the consumers and budget holders of biosurveillance enterprise.

DoD did not appear to have consolidated and accurate documentation in one place of all of the information systems, data sources, data collection frequencies, and outputs that comprise the current biosurveillance effort. This may have limited the study team's ability to fully assess the status and gaps in DoD biosurveillance.

Despite these limitations, the study team found sufficient evidence to offer evidence-based responses to the three tasks specified by OMB.

Responses to the Three OMB Tasks

This Study Responds to OMB's Three Tasks

- *Task 1: Identify a prioritized list of DoD biosurveillance programs, missions, desired outcomes, and associated performance measures and targets*
  - ➢ The highest-priority missions are force health protection > biological weapons defense > global health security
  - ➢ Desired outcomes: early warning/early detection, situational awareness, better decision making, forecasting impacts
  - ➢ Prioritization of strategic missions suggests that the highest-priority biosurveillance programs should be the 21 that address force health protection, followed by the one that addresses biological weapons defense (but not force health protection), and then the seven programs that address only global health security

- *Task 2: Evaluate how the current array of program assets contributes to achieving the prioritized missions*
  - ➢ DoD biosurveillance supports the three strategic missions and four outcomes
  - ➢ More near-real-time analysis and better internal and external integration will enhance the performance and value of DoD biosurveillance to DoD decision makers, especially for current situational awareness
  - ➢ Improvements are needed in key enablers, including the need for explicit doctrine/policy, efficient organization and governance, increased staffing, and improved facilities for AFHSC

- *Task 3: Assess whether the current funding system is appropriate and how it can be improved to ensure stable funding*
  - ➢ There is no funding system for the enterprise, and the multiple funding systems that invest in the enterprise at the moment would likely benefit from an organizing mechanism with the authority to manage and control funds to meet enterprise goals
  - ➢ Interim guidance issued by Deputy Secretary of Defense on June 13, 2013, is significant: (a) first policy to explicitly address biosurveillance; (b) adopts the definition from the National Strategy for Biosurveillance; (c) calls for development of a DoD Directive for biosurveillance; (d) specifies tasks for DoD implementation of the Strategy

Biosurveillance, as any health-related surveillance, is considered a cornerstone of public (i.e., population) health and an extremely cost-effective investment. Absent formal cost-effectiveness analysis of the DoD biosurveillance enterprise, it is nonetheless reasonable to conclude that modest marginal investments toward a more integrated and efficient DoD biosurveillance enterprise will yield substantial returns in health, economic, and global health security terms.

This study responds to the OMB's three tasks:

- Task 1: Identify a prioritized list of DoD biosurveillance programs, missions, desired outcomes, and associated performance measures and targets.

  - Based on U.S. statutory authority, the highest-priority missions are force health protection and biological weapons defense; global health security is a third priority, based on national policy and U.S. government international obligations.
  - Desired biosurveillance outcomes are early warning and early detection, situational awareness, improved decision making, and forecast of impacts.
  - Programs and measures that address priority missions, force health protection in particular, and desired outcomes should be prioritized over those that do not do so

- Task 2: Evaluate how the current array of program assets contributes to achieving the prioritized missions.

  - DoD biosurveillance programs contribute to all three strategic-level missions and all four desired outcomes.

- More near-real-time analysis and better internal and external integration will enhance the performance and value of DoD biosurveillance to DoD decision makers, especially for current situational awareness.
- Improvements are needed in key enablers, including the need for explicit doctrine/policy, efficient organization and governance, and increased staffing and improved facilities for AFHSC.

- <u>Task 3</u>: Assess whether the current funding system is appropriate and how it can be improved to ensure stable funding.

  - There is no funding system for the enterprise, and the multiple funding systems that invest in the enterprise at the moment would likely benefit from an organizing mechanism with the authority to manage and control funds to meet enterprise goals.
  - Interim guidance issued by the Deputy Secretary of Defense on June 13, 2013, is significant because it is the first policy to explicitly address biosurveillance; it adopts the definition from the National Strategy for Biosurveillance, calls for development of a DoDD for biosurveillance, and specifies tasks for DoD implementation of the Strategy.

Appendix A. Documents Reviewed

FEDERAL LEGISLATION

1. 10 U.S.C. - Section 142, *Assistant to the Secretary of Defense for Nuclear and Chemical and Biological Defense Programs*.
2. 32 CFR - Title 32, "National Defense."
3. 50 U.S.C - Section 1522, "Conduct of Chemical and Biological Defense Program."
4. 50 U.S.C - Section 1523, "Annual Report on Chemical and Biological Warfare Defense."
5. 42 U.S.C. 5121 et seq. Chapter 68."Disaster Relief."

NATIONAL POLICY/STRATEGY/GUIDANCE

1. Centers for Disease Control and Prevention, "National Biosurveillance Strategy for Human Health, Version 2.0," February 2010.
   http://www.cdc.gov/osels/pdf/NBSHH_v2.pdf
2. Department of Health and Human Services, *National Health Security Strategy of the United States of America*, December 2009.
   http://www.phe.gov/Preparedness/planning/authority/nhss/strategy/Documents/nhss-final.pdf
3. Department of Homeland Security, "National Preparedness Goal," September 2011.
   https://www.fema.gov/pdf/prepared/npg.pdf
4. Homeland Security Presidential Directive 10, "Biodefense for the 21st Century," April 28, 2004.
   https://www.hsdl.org/?collection/stratpol&id=pd&pid=gwb
5. Homeland Security Presidential Directive 21, "Public Health and Medical Preparedness," October 18, 2007. https://www.hsdl.org/?collection/stratpol&id=pd&pid=gwb
6. Presidential Decision Directive 2, *National Strategy for Countering Biological Threats*, November 2009.
7. Presidential Decision Directive NSTC-7, "Emerging Infectious Diseases," June 12, 1996.
8. Presidential Policy Directive 8, "National Preparedness," March 30, 2011.
9. White House, *National Strategy for Biosurveillance*, July 2012.
   http://www.whitehouse.gov/sites/default/files/National_Strategy_for_Biosurveillance_July_2012.pdf
10. White House, "Memorandum: Fiscal Year 2015 Budget Guidance for Countering Biological Threats Resource Priorities," June 27, 2013.
11. White House, *National Security Strategy*, May 2010.
    http://www.whitehouse.gov/sites/default/files/rss_viewer/national_security_strategy.pdf
12. White House, *National Security Strategy*, March 2006.
    http://georgewbush-whitehouse.archives.gov/nsc/nss/2006/index.html
13. White House National Security Staff, Emerging Pandemic Threats Sub-Interagency Policy Committee, "Promoting Global Health Security: Guidance and Principles for U.S. Government Departments and Agencies to Strengthen IHR Core Capacities Internationally," June 2011. (not available to the public)

DoD DOCTRINE/POLICY/GUIDANCE

1. Chairman of the Joint Chiefs of Staff Instruction (CJCSI) 3112.01B, "Joint Biological Warfare Defense Capabilities," November 2, 2012.
2. Department of Defense, "Implementation Plan for the National Strategy for Biosurveillance," February 15, 2013.
3. Department of Defense, "Memorandum: Interim Guidance for Implementing the National Strategy for Biosurveillance," January 2013.
4. Department of Defense Directive 2060.02, "Department of Defense (DoD) Combating Weapons of Mass Destruction (WMD) Policy," April 19, 2007.
5. Department of Defense Directive 3025.18, "Defense Support of Civil Authorities (DSCA)," December 29, 2010.
6. Department of Defense Directive 4715.1E, "Environment, Safety, and Occupational Health (ESOH)," March 19, 2005.
7. Department of Defense Directive 5105.21, "Defense Intelligence Agency (DIA)," March 18, 2008.
8. Department of Defense Directive 5105.62, "Defense Threat Reduction Agency," April 24, 2013.
9. Department of Defense Directive 5124.02, "Under Secretary of Defense for Personnel and Readiness (USD[P&R])," June 23, 2008.
10. Department of Defense Directive 5134.01, "Under Secretary of Defense for Acquisition, Technology, and Logistics (USD[AT&L])," April 1, 2008.
11. Department of Defense Directive 5134.08, "Assistant Secretary of Defense for Nuclear, Chemical, and Biological Defense Programs (ASD[NCB])," February14, 2013.
12. Department of Defense Directive 5136.01, "Assistant Secretary of Defense for Health Affairs (ASD[HA])," June 4, 2008.
13. Department of Defense Directive 5143.01, "Under Secretary of Defense for Intelligence (USD[I])," November 23, 2005.
14. Department of Defense Directive 5160.05E, "Roles and Responsibilities Associated with the Chemical and Biological Defense (CBD) Program (CBDP)," October 9, 2008.
15. Department of Defense Directive 5240.01, "DoD Intelligence Activities," August 27, 2007.
16. Department of Defense Directive 6205.02E. "Policy and Program for Immunizations to Protect the Health of Service Members and Military Beneficiaries," September 19, 2006.
17. Department of Defense Instruction 6200.03, "Public Health Emergency Management within the Department of Defense," June 2012.
18. Department of Defense Directive 6200.04, "Force Health Protection (FHP)," April 2007.
19. Department of Defense Directive 6490.02E, "Comprehensive Health Surveillance," February 8, 2012.
20. Department of Defense Instruction 6420.01, "National Center for Medical Intelligence (NCMI)," March 20, 2009.
21. Department of Defense Instruction 6440.03, "Department of Defense Laboratory Network (DLN)," June 2011.
22. Department of Defense Instruction 6490.03, "Deployment Health," August 11, 2006.
23. Joint Publication 1-02, *Department of Defense Dictionary of Military and Associated Terms*, April 2013.

24. Office of the Secretary of Defense, "Memorandum: Interim Guidance for Implementing the National Strategy for Biosurveillance," June 13, 2013.

25. Office of the Secretary of Defense, "Memorandum: Establishing an Armed Forces Health Surveillance Center," February 26, 2008.

26. Office of the Secretary of Defense, "Memorandum: Policy for DoD Global, Laboratory-Based Influenza Surveillance," February 3, 1999.

AFHSC-SPECIFIC DOCUMENTS

1. Armed Forces Health Surveillance Center, AFHSC Base Funding TMA MEDCOM, July 15, 2013.

2. Armed Forces Health Surveillance Center, Dr. Rohit Chitale, "Division of Integrated Biosurveillance," (PowerPoint Presentation) May 16, 2013.

3. Armed Forces Health Surveillance Center, "(EA) Comprehensive Resource Review," April 19, 2013.

4. Armed Forces Health Surveillance Center, "Biosurveillance Program Objectives Memorandum, 8 of 8 Priorities," 2013, for POM 2015. (not available to the public)

5. Armed Forces Health Surveillance Center, "DMSS Structure and Functional Relationships, All DoD Beneficiaries," April 2013.

6. Armed Forces Health Surveillance Center, "Recurrent Reports Distribution," April 16, 2013.

7. Armed Forces Health Surveillance Center, Division of Data Management and Technical Support, "DMSS Interfaces," March 14, 2013.

8. Armed Forces Health Surveillance Center, Strategic Plan for Fiscal Years 2013-2015, January 28, 2013.

9. Armed Forces Health Surveillance Center, "HA-NCB MOU Operational Plan Execution: AFHSC Requirements," March 17, 2013.

10. Armed Forces Health Surveillance Center, "AFHSC Annual Report - Division of Integrated Biosurveillance (DRAFT)," January 2013.

11. Armed Forces Health Surveillance Center, "FY13 AFHSC GEIS funded partners by service lab," January 2013.

12. Armed Forces Health Surveillance Center, "AFHSC Publications FY2012," 2013.

13. Armed Forces Health Surveillance Center, "AFHSC Epidemiologic and Analysis Recurrent and Ad Hoc Reports," 2013.

14. Armed Forces Health Surveillance Center, "Ad Hoc Requests 2012," 2013.

15. Armed Forces Health Surveillance Center, Dr. Rohit Chitale, "Biosurveillance: An Interagency Perspective," September 7, 2012.

16. Armed Forces Health Surveillance Center, "Armed Forces Reportable Medical Events Guidelines and Case Definitions," March 2012. http://www.afhsc.mil/viewDocument?file=TriService_CaseDefDocs/ArmedForcesGuidlinesFinal14Mar12.pdf

17. Armed Forces Health Surveillance Center, "A DoD Biosurveillance Capability: Moving Forward on Implementation," April 16, 2012.

18. Armed Forces Health Surveillance Center, "U.S. Department of Defense: Integrated Biosurveillance Capability ", February 23, 2012. (not available to the public)

19. Armed Forces Health Surveillance Center, "The U.S. Department of Defense: Integrated Biosurveillance Capability, Guidance for Biosurveillance and the AFHSC Involvement," February 13, 2012.

20. Armed Forces Health Surveillance Center, "Armed Forces Health Surveillance Center Fiscal Year 2011 Report," 2011.
http://www.afhsc.mil/viewDocument?file=AFHSC_AnnualReport_WEB.pdf

21. Armed Forces Health Surveillance Center, David Blazes, "Global Emerging Infections Surveillance and Response System (GEIS) Electronic Surveillance Initiatives," September 2010.
http://www.tatrc.org/conferences/ata_midyear_10/ppt/Blazes_ATA_MidYear_Sept10.pdf

22. Armed Forces Health Surveillance Center, "AFHSC CONOPS (DRAFT)," January 23, 2009.

23. Department of the Army, "Memorandum: Urgent Need to Acquire Additional Leased Space at the 11800 Tech Road Bldg., Silver Spring, MD or another Building for Consolidating Armed Forces Health Surveillance Center (Provisional) AFHSC (P)," July 7, 2008.

24. U.S. Army Center for Health Promotion and Preventive Medicine, "Memorandum: Government Leased or Owned Property for Consolidating the Armed Forces Health Surveillance Center (Provisional) in the National Capital Area," December 21, 2007.

DoD – OTHER

1. Bureau of Medicine and Surgery Instruction (BUMEDINST) 6220.12B, "Medical Surveillance and Notifiable Event Reporting," February 12, 2009.
http://www.med.navy.mil/sites/nmcphc/Documents/policy-and-instruction/bumed_inst_6220-12B.pdf

2. Defense Health Information Management System, "Medical Situational Awareness in Theater (MSAT) Fact Sheet."
http://dhims.health.mil/products/theater/msat.aspx

3. Defense Health Services Systems, "Electronic Surveillance System for the Early Notification of Community-Based Epidemics (ESSENCE) Fact Sheet," March 2013.
http://www.health.mil/MHSCIO/programs_products/DHSS/DHSS-Products/ESSENCE.aspx

4. Defense Threat Reduction Agency, "Cooperative Threat Reduction Program Fiscal Year (FY) 2014 Budget Estimates," 2013.
http://comptroller.defense.gov/defbudget/fy2014/budget_justification/pdfs/01_Operation_and_Maintenance/O_M_VOL_1_PART_2/CTR_OP-5.pdf . (accessed 19 June 2013).

5. Department of Defense, "Memorandum of Understanding between the U.S. Department of Defense Office of the Assistant Secretary of Defense for Nuclear, Chemical, and Biological Defense Programs and U.S. Department of Defense Office of the Assistant Secretary of Defense for Health Affairs," July 10, 2012.

6. Department of Defense, "Department of Defense Agency Financial Report for FY 2012."
http://comptroller.defense.gov/afr/fy2012/3-Financial_Section.pdf (accessed 13 June 2013).

7. Department of Defense, "Fiscal Year (FY) 2014 President's Budget Submission, Chemical Biological Defense Program, Justification Book Volume 4 of 4: Research, Development, Test & Evaluation, Defense-Wide," April 2013. http://comptroller.defense.gov/

8. Department of Defense, "Fiscal Year (FY) 2014 President's Budget Submission, Defense Health Program," April 2013.
    http://comptroller.defense.gov/

9. Department of Defense, "Fiscal Year (FY) 2014 Budget RDT&E Programs (R-1) – Unclassified." April 2013, D-18.
    http://comptroller.defense.gov/defbudget/fy2014/fy2014_r1.pdf

10. DHA Public Health sub Work Group, "Health Surveillance SME Team Brief 1," March 28, 2013.

11. DHA Public Health sub Work Group, "Public Health sub Work Group briefing part 1- overview, opportunities for improvement," March 28, 2013.

12. DHA Public Health sub Work Group, "Public Health sub Work Group briefing part 2- quantifying opportunities for improvement," April 23, 2013.

13. DHA Public Health sub Work Group, "Public Health sub Work Group briefing part 3- future state structures," May 16, 2013.

14. Joint Program Executive Office for Chemical and Biological Defense, "Joint Biological Agent Identification and Diagnostic System (JBAIDS) Fact Sheet," March 7, 2012.
    https://jacks.jpeocbd.army.mil/Jacks/Public/FactSheetProvider.ashx?productId=344

15. Joint Program Executive Office for Chemical and Biological Defense, "NBC Contamination Avoidance," September 19, 2012.
    http://www.jpeocbd.osd.mil/packs/DocHandler.ashx?DocID=13074

16. Joint Staff/J-8, "Joint DOTmLPF-P Change Recommendation for Biosurveillance, Version 1.9.3 (DRAFT)," March 27, 2013. (not available to the public)

17. Office of the Secretary of Defense, "Report on Department of Defense Biosurveillance: Roles, Missions, and Functions," August 2011.

18. Office of the Secretary of Defense, "Action Memo: Interim Guidance for Implementation of the National Strategy for Biosurveillance," May 14, 2013. (not available to the public)

19. Offices of the Assistant Secretaries of Defense for Health Affairs and Nuclear, Chemical, and Biological Defense Programs, "HA-NCB Memorandum of Understanding Operational Plan," February 26, 2013.

20. OPNAV Instruction (OPNAVINST) 6100.3, "Deployment Health Assessment (DHA) Process," January 9, 2012.
    http://www.med.navy.mil/sites/nmcphc/Documents/epi-data-center/OPNAV-6100.3.pdf

U.S. GOVERNMENT - OTHER

1. Centers for Disease Control and Prevention, "Updated Guidelines for Evaluating Public Health Surveillance Systems: Recommendations from the Guidelines Working Group," *MMWR,* Vol. 50(No. RR-13), 2001.

2. Centers for Disease Control and Prevention, "Public Health Preparedness Capabilities: National Standards for State and Local Planning," March 2011.
    http://www.cdc.gov/phpr/capabilities/ (accessed 19 June 2013).

3. U.S. Government Accountability Office, "Biosurveillance: Developing a Collaboration Strategy Is Essential to Fostering Interagency Data and Resource Sharing (GAO-10-171)," Washington, DC, December 18, 2009.

4. U.S. Government Accountability Office, "Biosurveillance: Efforts to Develop a National Biosurveillance Capability Need a National Strategy and a Designated Leader (GAO 10-645)," Washington, DC, June 30, 2010.

INTERNATIONAL

1. World Health Organization, *International Health Regulations (2005), 2nd ed*, Geneva, 2008.
   http://whqlibdoc.who.int/publications/2008/9789241580410_eng.pdf
2. World Health Organization, "IHR Core Capacity Monitoring Framework: Checklist and Indicators for Monitoring Progress in the Development of IHR Core Capacities in States Parties," June 2012.
   http://www.who.int/ihr/checklist/en/

PUBLISHED PAPERS

1. Blazes, D. L., J. L. Bondarenko, R. L. Burke, et. al,, "Contributions of the Global Emerging Infections Surveillance and Response System Network to Global Health Security in 2011," *The Army Medical Department Journal*, No. PB 8-13-4/5/6, April–June 2013, pp. 7–18.
2. Camm, F., and B. M. Stecher, *Analyzing the Operation of Performance-Based Accountability Systems for Public Services* (TR-853). Santa Monica, Calif.: RAND Corporation, 2010.
   http://www.rand.org/pubs/technical_reports/TR853.html
3. Cox, K. L., "Global Influenza Surveillance in the U.S. Military," paper presented at RTO HFM Symposium on NATO Medical Surveillance and Response, Research and Technology Opportunities and Options, Budapest, Hungary, April 19–21, 2004.
4. Greenfield, V., V. Williams, and E. Eiseman, *Using Logic Models for Strategic Planning and Evaluation: Application to the National Center for Injury Prevention and Control* (TR-370), Santa Monica, Calif.: RAND Corporation, 2006.
   http://www.rand.org/pubs/technical_reports/TR370.html
5. Ijaz, K., E. Kasowski, R. R. Arthur, F. J. Angulo, and S. F. Dowell, "International Health Regulations: What Gets Measured Gets Done," *Emerging Infectious Diseases,* Vol. 18, No. 7, July 2012, pp. 1054–1057.
   http://www.ncbi.nlm.nih.gov/pubmed/22709593
6. Institute of Medicine, *The Future of the Public's Health in the 21st Century*, Washington, DC: National Academies Press, 2003.
7. MacIntosh, V. H., "Enhancing Influenza Surveillance Using Electronic Surveillance System for the Early Notification of Community-Based Epidemics (ESSENCE)," paper presented at RTO HFM Symposium on NATO Medical Surveillance and Response, Research and Technology Opportunities and Options, Budapest, Hungary, April 19–21, 2004.
8. McNabb, S.J. N., S. Chungong, M. Ryan, T. Wuhib, P. Nusbuga, W. Alemu, V. Carande-Kulis, and G. Rodier, "Conceptual Framework of Public Health Surveillance and Action and Its Application in Health Sector Reform," *BMC Public Health,* Vol. 2, No. 2, 2002.
   http://www.biomedcentral.com/1471-2458/2/2
9. Moore, M., "The Global Dimensions of Public Health Preparedness and Implications for US Action," *American Journal of Public Health*, Vol. 102, No. 6, 2012, p. e1–7.
   http://www.ncbi.nlm.nih.gov/pubmed/22515870
10. Moore, M., D.J. Dausey, B. Phommasack, S. Touch, G. Lu, S. Lwin Nyein, K. Ungchusak, N.D. Vung, and M.K. Oo, "Sustainability of Sub-Regional Disease Surveillance Networks," *Global Health Governance*, Vol. V, No. 2, Spring 2012.
    http://www.ncbi.nlm.nih.gov/pmc/articles/PMC3557953/

11. Moore, M., E. Chan, N. Lurie, A. G. Schaefer, D. M. Varda, and J. A. Zambrano, "Strategies to Improve Global Influenza Surveillance: A Decision Tool for Policymakers," *BMC Public Health*, Vol. 8, 2008, p. 186. http://www.ncbi.nlm.nih.gov/pubmed/18507852

12. Moore, M., E. Eisemann, G. Fischer, S. Olmsted, P. Sama, and J. Zambrano, *Harnessing Full Value from the DoD Serum Repository and the Defense Medical Surveillance System* (MG875), Santa Monica, Calif.: RAND Corporation, 2010. http://www.rand.org/pubs/monographs/MG875.html

13. Nsubuga, P., M. E. White, S. B. Thacker, M. A. Anderson, S. B. Blount, C. V. Broome, T. Chiller, V. Espitia, R. Imtiaz, D. Sosin, D.F. Stroup, R.V. Tauxe. "Chapter 53 - Public Health Surveillance: A Tool for Targeting and Monitoring Interventions," in D. T. Jamison et al., eds., *Disease Control Priorities in Developing Countries. 2nd ed.* Washington, DC: World Bank, 2006.

14. Owens, A. B., L. C. Canas, K. L. Russell, J. S. Neville, J. A. Pavlin, V. H. MacIntosh, G. C. Gray, and J. C. Gaydos, "Department of Defense Global Laboratory-Based Influenza Surveillance: 1998–2005," *American Journal of Preventive Medicine,* Vol. 37, No. 3, 2009, pp. 235–241. www.ncbi.nlm.nih.gov/pubmed/19666159

15. Peake, J. B., J. S. Morrison, M. M. Ledgerwood, and S. E. Gannon, *The Defense Department's Enduring Contributions to Global Health: The Future of the U.S. Army and Navy Overseas Medical Research Laboratories*, Washington, DC: Center for Strategic and International Studies, June 2011.

16. PricewaterhouseCoopers, "Operationalizing the DoD Biosurveillance Enterprise: Integrating DoD BSV Capabilities and Developing an Implementation Roadmap," April 2013.

17. Sanchez, J. L., "Global Emerging Infections Surveillance and Response in the U.S. Military," Presented at the Global Health Pathway Tropical & Travel Medicine Seminar, October 24, 2012. http://www.globalhealth.umn.edu/prod/groups/med/@pub/@med/@dom/@global/documents/article/med_article_416866.pdf

18. Shelton, S. R., A. W. McLees, K. Mumford, and C. Thomas, "Building Performance-Based Accountability With Limited Empirical Evidence: Performance Measurement for Public Health Preparedness," *Disaster Medicine and Public Health Preparedness*, Vol. 0, No. 0, 2013.

19. Thacker, S. B., "Historical Development," in S. T. Teutsch and R. E. Churchill, eds., *Principles and Practice of Public Health Surveillance*, New York: Oxford University Press, 2000.

20. Witt, C. J., A. L. Richards, P. M. Masuoka et al., "The AFHSC-Division of GEIS Operations Predictive Surveillance Program: A Multidisciplinary Approach for the Early Detection and Response to Disease Outbreaks," *BMC Public Health,* Vol. 11 Suppl 2, March 4, 2011. www.biomedcentral.com/1471-2458/11/S2/S10

Appendix B. Mission Authorities

Table B.1. Authoritative Sources of Different DoD Missions

Mission	Text	Document
Force health protection	Full Implementation of **Medical Readiness Tracking and Health Surveillance Program** and Force Health Protection and Readiness Program (a) The Secretary of Defense, in conjunction with the Secretaries of the military departments, shall take such actions are as necessary to ensure that the Army, Navy, Air Force, and Marine Corps fully implement at all levels - (1) the Medical Readiness Tracking and Health Surveillance Program under this title...; and (2) the Force Health Protection and Readiness Program of the DoD (relating to the prevention of injury and illness and the reduction of disease and noncombat injury threats).	U.S. Code Title 10, Chapter 55
Force health protection	4.3. The **DoD Components** shall **implement programs** and processes that **promote and sustain a healthy and fit force**, prevent injury and illness, **protect the force from health hazards**, and deliver the best possible medical and rehabilitative care to the sick and injured anywhere in the world. (p. 2)	DoDD 6200.04 Force Health Protection
Force health protection	4.(a) "It is DoD policy that: **Comprehensive health surveillance is an important element of force health protection programs** to promote, protect and restore the physical and mental health of DoD personnel throughout their military service and employment, both in garrison and during deployment..." This Directive: ...Establishes the Armed Forces Health Surveillance Center (AFHSC) as the single source for DoD-level health surveillance information. (p. 1)	DoDD 6490.02E Comprehensive Health Surveillance
Global health security	The mission of DoD will be expanded to include support of **global surveillance**, training, research and response to emerging infectious disease threats. DoD will strengthen its global disease reduction efforts through: centralized coordination, improved preventive health programs and epidemiological capabilities, and enhanced involvement with military treatment facilities and United States and overseas laboratories.	PPD NSTC 7 Emerging Infectious Diseases
Global health security	NCMI is the DoD lead activity for the production of medical intelligence and will **prepare and coordinate integrated, all-source intelligence** for the Department of Defense and other government and international organizations **on foreign health threats** and other medical issues to protect U.S. interests worldwide. (p. 2)	DoDI 6420.01NCMI
Biological weapons defense	(b) "The Secretary of Defense shall....(1) Assign responsibility for overall coordination and integration of the chemical and **biological warfare defense program** and the chemical and biological medical defense program to a single office within the Office of the Secretary of Defense. (2) Take those actions necessary to ensure close and continuous coordination between (a) the chemical and biological warfare defense program, and (b) the chemical and biological medical defense program. (3) Exercise oversight over the chemical and biological defense program through the Defense Acquisition Board process."	U.S. Code Title 50, Section 1522 Conduct of Chemical and Biological Defense Program
Biological weapons defense	4. "It is policy that the **DoD will combat WMD** to dissuade, deter, and defeat those who seek to harm the United States, its citizens, its Armed forces, and its friends and allies through WMD use or threat of use, while maintaining the ability to respond to and mitigate the effects of WMD use, and to restore deterrence."	DoDD 2060.02 Combating Weapons of Mass Destruction

97

Mission	Text	Document
Biological weapons defense	The mission of DTRA is to safeguard the United States and its allies from weapons of mass destruction (WMD) threats globally. (p. 1)The Director, DTRA: Supports DoD collaboration with departments and agencies across the U.S. government to **enhance the capacity of other nations to counter WMD**. (p. 10)	DoDD 5105.62 Defense Threat Reduction Agency
Public health & medical	(Medical) The USD(P&R) shall develop policies, plans, and programs for Health and medical affairs to provide health services and support to members of the Armed Forces during military operations. (p. 3)	DoDD 5124.02 Under Secretary of Defense for Personnel and Readiness (USD[P&R])
Public health & medical	The ASD(HA) is the principal advisor to the Secretary of Defense and the USD(P&R) for all DoD health policies, programs, and force health protection activities. The ASD(HA) shall ensure the effective execution of the Department's **medical mission, providing and maintaining readiness for medical services and support to members of the Armed Forces**, including during military operations (p. 3)	DoDD 5136.01Assistant Secretary of Defense for Health Affairs (ASD[HA])
International collaboration & capacity building	The Director, DTRA: Supports DoD collaboration with departments and agencies across the U.S. government to **enhance the capacity of other nations to counter WMD**. (p. 10)	DoDD 5105.62 Defense Threat Reduction Agency
Countering WMD	The mission of DTRA is to safeguard the United States and its allies from weapons of mass destruction (WMD) threats globally. (p. 1)	DoDD 5105.62 Defense Threat Reduction Agency
Health/ biosurveillance	This Directive: Establishes the Armed Forces Health Surveillance Center (AFHSC) as the single source for DoD-level health surveillance information. (pg 1)	DoDD 6490.02E Comprehensive Health Surveillance
Health/ biosurveillance	The Heads of the DoD Components shall: b. **Provide appropriate medical support and training, equipment, and supplies to implement health** and medical **surveillance** within and, where applicable, jointly across their respective Components. (p. 6)	DoDD 6490.02E Comprehensive Health Surveillance
Health/ biosurveillance	The USD(AT&L) shall, consistent with References (e) and DoDD 5134.01 (Reference (l)), **align the environment, safety, and occupational and environmental health programs with** comprehensive **health surveillance activities.** (p. 6)	DoDD 6490.02E Comprehensive Health Surveillance
Health/ biosurveillance	It is DoD policy that: Comprehensive, continuous, and consistent **health surveillance shall be conducted by the Military Services** to implement early intervention and control strategies using technologies, practices, and procedures in a consistent manner across the DoD Components pursuant to this Directive. (p. 2)	DoDD 6490.02E Comprehensive Health Surveillance
R&D	The Director, DTRA integrates assigned CWMD activities and tasks across the DoD, as appropriate. In this capacity, the Director: Manages and oversees DTRA research, development, test, and evaluation (RDT&E) and acquisition needed to support DoD mission areas, this includes support of OSD strategic and tactical systems acquisition oversight of DoD; Assists the ASD(NCB) to develop a comprehensive research, development, and acquisition strategy to combat WMD, consistent with References(d) and (h), and in support of DoDD 5160.05E (Reference (i))	DoDD 5105.62 Defense Threat Reduction Agency
Medical intelligence	It is DoD policy that: **NCMI is the DoD lead activity for the production of medical intelligence and will** prepare and coordinate integrated, all-source intelligence for the Department of Defense and other government and international organizations on foreign health threats and other medical issues to protect U.S. interests worldwide. (p. 2)	DoDI 6420.01 National Center for Medical Intelligence

Appendix C. DoD Biosurveillance Systems and Assets

Table C.1. Characteristics of Key DoD Biosurveillance Systems

Mission(s) Served DoD Owner System	Link to AFHSC	Coverage/Completeness of Populations	Coverage/Completeness of Events Monitored	Quality/Accuracy	Timeliness (Frequency)
Force health protection **Air Force/U.S. Air Force School of Aerospace Medicine (USAFSAM)** Air Force Reportable Events Surveillance System (**AFRESS – II;** soon to transition to Disease Reporting System internet - *DRSi*)	DMSS	All Air Force and beneficiaries reportable medical events (RMEs); All deployed active duty and Air Force reserves before and twice after return from deployment (Health Assessment)	Air Force RMEs: 66 conditions with standardized case definitions; Health assessment questionnaires	Clinical diagnosis, lab-confirmed as warranted; self report	*Data collection*: Daily *Data feeds*: Weekly *Data analysis*: (same as Army and Navy DRSi)
Force health protection **Army/Medical Research and Materiel Command (MRMC)** Armed Forces Medical Examiners System (**AFMES**) – houses the DNA Identification Lab (AFDIL) and the DoD Medical Mortality Registry, which contains the mortality data	DMSS	Active duty and activated reserves	Casualty data	Identifies deaths due to unexplained circumstances or infectious disease and evaluates mortality trends and risk factors; Determines definitive diagnosis based on medical records, autopsy reports, and pathological reports	*Data collection*: Daily *Data feeds*: Monthly *Data analysis*: Based on mortality requests

99

Mission(s) Served DoD Owner System	Link to AFHSC	Coverage/Completeness of Populations	Coverage/Completeness of Events Monitored	Quality/Accuracy	Timeliness (Frequency)
Force health protection **Army/USAPHC** Acute Respiratory Disease Surveillance Program	GEIS	Army basic training populations	Acute respiratory diseases	Clinically based report; added to the AFHSC Weekly Respiratory Report	*Data collection*: Daily *Data feeds*: Weekly *Data analysis*: Weekly
Global health security **USD(AT&L)/JPEO** Biosurveillance Ecosystem (**BSV-E**) (NOT YET FIELDED)	DIB	Peru, Kenya/Uganda, Northern Australia, Cambodia, Thailand	Malaria, dengue, *Burkholderia pseudomallei*	When completed will come from various sources; moderate to high quality	Monthly at first, then daily
Force health protection **ASD(HA)/TMA** Defense Health Services Systems (**DHSS**)	DMSS	All active duty Service members, including visits to 260 DoD healthcare facilities world wide	Clinical visits (inpatient and outpatient) and associated diagnostic tests and pharmacy transactions; medical readiness (e.g., immunizations)	High - definitive	*Data collection*: Daily *Data feeds*: Daily – CAPER (outpatient), HL-7 (lab) Monthly – Master patient index, SIDR (inpatient), TED_NI, TED_I *Data analysis*: Analysis using the DMSS is occurring on many products every day, dependent on subject and requests

100

Mission(s) Served DoD Owner System	Link to AFHSC	Coverage/Completeness of Populations	Coverage/Completeness of Events Monitored	Quality/Accuracy	Timeliness (Frequency)
Force health protection **AFHSC** Defense Medical Surveillance System (**DMSS**) *Data feeds not listed separately below include:* - **ADMF** (Active Duty Master File) - personnel data - **ASIMS** (Aeromedicine Services Info. Mgt. Systems) - deployment assessments - **CDD_Army,** **CDD_MEPS, CDD_Navy** (Centers for Disease Detection - HIV serology data) - **DEERS** (Defense Enrollment Eligibility System) – immunizations - **LIMS** (Laboratory Info. Mgt. System) - HIV serology data	AFHSC owner	All active duty Service members throughout their careers	Personnel data; deployment data; casualty data; clinical visits (inpatient & outpatient) and associated diagnostic tests and pharmacy transactions; medical readiness (e.g., immunizations); theater medical encounters; reportable medical events; deployment health assessments; Military Entrance Processing Station screening	Definitive DoD data sources; clinical diagnosis, lab-confirmed as warranted; lab-based screening	*Data collection*: Daily *Data feeds*: Daily - outpatient, lab tests, pharmacy, immunizations, deployment health assessments; Weekly - reportable events, HIV serology; Monthly - personnel, casualty, deployment, inpatients (SIDR), MEPS *Data analysis*: Daily (dependent on subject and requests)
Force health protection **DoD/MHS** Defense Occupational and Environmental Health Readiness System (**DOEHRS**)	Direct query to USAPHC/ Army Institute of Public Health	Occupational and Environmental Health Events on DoD installations worldwide	Analysis results of air, water, soil samples (e.g., non-potable water, contaminated soil, airborne chemicals, poisonous plants)	Dependent on the technician and thoroughness of completing the reports and uploading them into the DOEHRS database	*Data collection*: Daily *Data feeds*: Query directly; DOEHRS Data Warehouse Web access will come online in June 2013 to extract data feeds online *Data analysis*: Based on demand

101

Mission(s) Served DoD Owner System	Link to AFHSC	Coverage/Completeness of Populations	Coverage/Completeness of Events Monitored	Quality/Accuracy	Timeliness (Frequency)
Force health protection **Army/USAPHC** Deployment health assessments—Army Medical Department/Medical Protection System **(MEDPROS)**	DMSS	All deployed active duty and reserve Army, before and twice after return from deployment	Health assessment questionnaires	Self report	*Data collection*: Daily *Data feeds*: Daily *Data analysis*: Monthly (Health Assessment Report, PDHA/PDHRA Summary Reports)
Force health protection **Navy/Navy and Marine Corps Public Health Center (NMCPHC)** Deployment health assessments—Electronic Deployment Health Assessment database **(eDHA)**	DMSS	All deployed active duty and Navy reserves, before and twice after return from deployment	Health assessment questionnaires	Self report	*Data collection*: Daily *Data feeds*: Daily *Data analysis*: Monthly (same as preceding item for Army)

Mission(s) Served DoD Owner System	Link to AFHSC	Coverage/Completeness of Populations	Coverage/Completeness of Events Monitored	Quality/Accuracy	Timeliness (Frequency)
Force health protection **Army/USAPHC** **DRSi**	DMSS	All Army and dependents	Army RMEs: 66 conditions with standardized case definitions	Clinical diagnosis, lab-confirmed as warranted	*Data collection*: Daily *Data feeds*: Weekly *Data analysis*: *Daily* - Service liaisons and analysts review and use information daily; *More than weekly* - Ad hoc reports are requested, reviewed, approved and assigned to analysts three times per week *Weekly* - Analysis often carried out over several days to produce weekly reports; weekly and other recurrent reports involve substantial quality assurance to validate results
Global health security **GEIS/Ministry of Health (MoH)** Early Warning Outbreak Response System **(EWORS)**	GEIS	Foreign national populations in Indonesia	Syndromic surveillance for disease outbreaks - customized for the MoH	Hospital and clinic visits	*Data collection*: Daily *Data feeds*: MoH *Data analysis*: Locally at MoH

103

Mission(s) Served / DoD Owner / System	Link to AFHSC	Coverage/Completeness of Populations	Coverage/Completeness of Events Monitored	Quality/Accuracy	Timeliness (Frequency)
Force health protection **DoD/MHS** Electronic Surveillance System for the Early Notification of Community-based Epidemics (**ESSENCE**)	Online review	Collects from all permanent U.S. military medical treatment facilities around the world (CONUS, OCONUS)	Syndromes: Respiratory, fever, gastrointestinal, dermatological-hemorrhagic, dermatological-infectious, neurological, coma	Pre-diagnosis; AFHSC reviews data as needed to validate information incorporated into the weekly communicable disease report	*Data collection*: 4x/day *Data feeds*: Daily *Data analysis*: Reviewed daily by Service PH centers and military treatment facilities (MTFs)
Global health security **State Dept, Army/WRAIR (Armed Forces Research Institute of Medical Sciences [AFRIMS], U.S. Army Medical Research Unit [USAMRU]-Kenya) NAMRU-2** Embassy Based Respiratory Surveillance	GEIS	U.S. Embassy-affiliated personnel in 46 countries receiving test kits via GEIS: Afghanistan, Australia, Bangladesh, Burma, Cambodia, Chile, China, Colombia, Egypt, El Salvador, Germany, Ghana, India, Indonesia, Iraq, Italy, Jordan, Kazakhstan, Kenya, South Korea, Kuwait, Laos, Malaysia, Mali, Mexico, Nepal, Nigeria, Pakistan, Peru, Philippines, Poland, Russia, Saudi Arabia, Senegal, Serbia, Singapore, South Africa, Sri Lanka, Sudan, Taiwan, Thailand, Turkey, United Kingdom, Venezuela, Vietnam, Zimbabwe	Respiratory infections	Symptom clusters	*Sample collection*: Seasonal *Data feeds*: RDD/Weekly *Data analysis*: As received through RDD; Quarterly reports input to GEIS

Mission(s) Served DoD Owner System	Link to AFHSC	Coverage/Completeness of Populations	Coverage/Completeness of Events Monitored	Quality/Accuracy	Timeliness (Frequency)
Force health protection, Global health security **Air Force/USAFSAM** Global DoD Lab Based Influenza Surveillance and Response System	GEIS/ DMSS through the AHLTA/ Composite Health Care System feeds	U.S. military at 83 sentinel sites at U.S. MTFs around the globe	Influenza and other respiratory disease outbreaks	Lab confirmed; weekly report added to AFHSC Weekly Respiratory Report	*Collection:* As appropriate during outbreaks-6 samples per week from each sentinel site; *Data feeds:* Daily via the Respiratory Disease Dashboard; AHLTA/ Composite Health Care System *Data analysis:* Weekly during influenza season; Epi Chiefs q2wks; Monthly Teleconference; Qtrly reports; Outbreaks: w/in 24 hours

105

Mission(s) Served DoD Owner System	Link to AFHSC	Coverage/Completeness of Populations	Coverage/Completeness of Events Monitored	Quality/Accuracy	Timeliness (Frequency)
Force health protection, Global health security **AFHSC** Global Emerging Infections Surveillance and Response System (**GEIS**)	(GEIS)	Foreign populations in approximately 75 countries (full listing in Appendix D)	Five GEIS pillars: (1) respiratory infections with an emphasis on avian and pandemic influenza, (2) gastrointestinal infections, (3) febrile and vector-borne infections, (4) antimicrobial resistance, and (5) sexually transmitted infections Geographic variation in some specific diseases, depending on local prevalence/relevance	Lab confirmation is non-systematic (based on funded proposals), but when performed, quality is excellent	*Data collection*: Project/program oriented *Data feeds*: Varies from <24 hours for unique findings to less frequent; specimen results <3wks, monthly/quarterly; frequency also dependent on agreement from host nation for data release *Data analysis*: Reports received weekly, quarterly and annually based surveillance type and project.
Force health protection **DoD/MHS** Medical Situational Awareness in Theater (**MSAT**)	DHSS/US TRANSCOM extracts TMDS/ TRAC3S/ JMEWS that feeds DMSS	OCONUS- Conflict - all deployed Service members on the 'ground', not shipboard	Diseases and injuries, physical and psychological trauma, patient tracking, chemical and biological threats, environmental and occupational health, intelligence, medical command and control data, personnel, unit locations and weather.	Military Health System records of deployed Services; high quality and accuracy	*Data collection*: Daily *Data feeds*: Users need to query the system daily, weekly, monthly *Data analysis*: Daily

106

Mission(s) Served DoD Owner System	Link to AFHSC	Coverage/Completeness of Populations	Coverage/Completeness of Events Monitored	Quality/Accuracy	Timeliness (Frequency)
Force health protection, Global health security, Biological weapons defense **DIA/NCMI** National Center for Medical Intelligence (**NCMI**)/Infectious Disease Surveillance Analysis	DIB	Worldwide scope that includes daily monitoring of approximately 165 countries	Daily monitoring of 70–80 diseases of military relevance; nature of countries' blood supplies; capacity of countries' medical system; capacity of medical defense facilities; socio-political and environmental factors	Finished intelligence products that typically reflect early/incomplete data	_Data collection_: Daily _Data feeds_: unclassified and classified reports _Data analysis_: Daily review of 70–80 diseases in 165 countries; others based on country and disease of choice
Force health protection **Navy/NMCPHC** Navy Disease Reporting System - internet (**NDRSi**)	DMSS	All Navy and Marine Corps active duty and dependents	(1) Navy/Marines RMEs: 66 conditions with standardized case definitions; (2) Standard Inpatient Data Record; (3) Standard Ambulatory Data Record; (4) lab, pharmacy transactions, pathology, radiology	Clinical diagnosis, lab-confirmed as warranted	_Data collection_: Daily _Data feeds_: Weekly _Data analysis_: (same as preceding item – Army DRSi)

Mission(s) Served DoD Owner System	Link to AFHSC	Coverage/Completeness of Populations	Coverage/Completeness of Events Monitored	Quality/Accuracy	Timeliness (Frequency)
Force health protection; Global health security; Biological weapons defense *(based on government grants)* **Army/WRAIR** **Navy/NMRC** **Air Force/USAFSAM** **OCONUS labs** *Army OCONUS labs:* AFRIMS, USAMRU-Kenya, USAMRU-Georgia, Landstuhl Regional Medical Center, Brian Allgood Army Community Hospital *Navy OCONUS labs:* NAMRU-2, NAMRU-3, NAMRU-6 *Army CONUS labs:* WRAIR, USAPHC *Navy/MC CONUS labs:* NHRC, NMRC, NMCPHC *Air Force CONUS lab:* USAFSAM	GEIS	CONUS- and OCONUS-based military beneficiaries; For GEIS work: Collaboration to support national surveillance in ~75 partner countries (see Appendix D, Table D.1)	Five GEIS pillars: (1) respiratory infections with an emphasis on avian and pandemic influenza, (2) gastrointestinal infections, (3) febrile and vector-borne infections, (4) antimicrobial resistance, and (5) sexually transmitted infections Geographic variation in some specific diseases, depending on local prevalence/relevance	Lab confirmation is non-systematic (based on funded proposals), but when performed, quality is excellent	*Data collection:* Project/program oriented *Data feeds:* Varies from <24 hours for unique findings to less frequent; specimen results <3wks, monthly/quarterly; frequency also dependent on agreement from host nation for data release *Data analysis:* Reports received weekly, quarterly and annually based surveillance type and project.

108

Mission(s) Served DoD Owner System	Link to AFHSC	Coverage/Completeness of Populations	Coverage/Completeness of Events Monitored	Quality/Accuracy	Timeliness (Frequency)
Global health security **DOS/OCONUS labs/MoH & MoD/AFHSC contract with JHU APL for development** Suite for Automated Global Electronic bioSurveillance (**SAGES**)	GEIS; through partner labs as host nation shares	Foreign national populations – [*N-6*] Peru (Civ-Mil); Nicaragua (MoD); [*N-2*] Cambodia (MoD); Malaysia (MoH); [*AFRIMS*] Thailand (Royal Thai Army); Philippines (MoH); [*USAMRU-Kenya*] Cameroon (MoD); Kenya (MoD); Uganda (MoD); [*Future*] El Salvador, Honduras, Guatemala, Belize, Costa Rica, Colombia, Dominican Republic.	Disease surveillance for compliance with IHR - specific diseases determined by the MoH or MoD priorities	Clinic visits	*Data collection*: Daily *Data feeds*: Country specific from daily to weekly feeds *Data analysis*: Performed within country MoH/MoD; some sharing with DoD partner labs

109

Table C.2. Characteristics of Key DoD Biosurveillance Laboratories and Other Assets

Mission(s) Served DoD Owner System	Link to AFHSC	Coverage/Completeness of Populations	Coverage/Completeness of Events Monitored	Quality/Accuracy	Timeliness (Frequency)
Global health security **USD(AT&L)/DTRA** Cooperative Biological Engagement Program **(CBEP)** Enables biosurveillance through host nation capacity/capability building (physical infrastructure and training)	CBEP owns no BSV data to link	20 countries: • Former Soviet Union (7): Armenia, Azerbaijan, Georgia, Kazakhstan, Russia, Ukraine, Uzbekistan • Southeast Asia (4): Cambodia, Lao PDR, Malaysia, Vietnam • Eastern and Southern Africa (5): Djibouti, Kenya, South Africa, Tanzania, Uganda • South Asia (2): India, Pakistan • Middle East (2): Afghanistan, Iraq	Especially Dangerous Pathogens (Group A Select Agents, potential pandemic pathogens) – baseline assessments rather than ongoing surveillance, and conducted by host nation (CBEP owns no data)	Typically lab-confirmed (CBEP programming supports lab capacity/capability development); however, CBEP does not own the data	Typically one-time studies to establish baseline epidemiology for endemic pathogens of interest
Force health protection, Global health security **Services** Defense Laboratories Network **(DLN)** - **USAMRIID, NMRC, USAFSAM, WRAIR, NHRC, others**	GEIS/indirectly to DMSS (via data feeds from Member's medical record)	Laboratories associated with CONUS and OCONUS MTFs – cover all military Service members, among others	Chemical, biological, radiological, and nuclear (CBRN) agents, infectious disease outbreaks, and other biological threats	Definitive laboratory testing (superb quality)	*Specimen collection:* Project oriented *Data feeds:* Within 24 hours for unique findings; monthly for routine data feeds *Lab/data analysis:* Reports: Epi Chiefs every two weeks; Monthly Teleconference; Quarterly reports; Outbreaks: w/in 24 hours

Mission(s) Served DoD Owner System	Link to AFHSC	Coverage/Completeness of Populations	Coverage/Completeness of Events Monitored	Quality/Accuracy	Timeliness (Frequency)
Force health protection **AFHSC** DoD Serum Repository **(DoDSR)**	AFHSC owner	All Service members, throughout their careers	Only routine testing is for HIV	Lab-confirmed diagnosis, mainly for antibodies (genetic material less reliably available in serum as presently stored)	*Specimen collection:* At MTF: Daily; Individual: every 2 years, pre/post deployment; AFHSC Pickup: every 7–8 weeks *Lab analysis:* Dependent on Research or Public Health Practice Studies; analysis performed by DoD and outside laboratories
Global health security **USD(AT&L)/DTRA** Electronic Integrated Disease Surveillance System **(EIDSS)**	Platform provided to host nation, which may choose to share data with DTRA or U.S. government (i.e., DoD owns no biosurveillance data)	(CBEP) All Former Soviet Union; Afghanistan, Pakistan, Iraq, Eastern and Southern Africa; Southeast Asia (EIDSS) Kazakhstan, Georgia, Azerbaijan, Armenia, Iraq	Clinically diagnosed information on infectious diseases that are considered WHO/Country determined notifiable diseases	Typically lab-confirmed (CBEP programming supports lab capacity/capability development)	*Data collection:* Daily *Data feeds:* Controlled locally by MoH *Data analysis:* Performed locally by MoH as they produce weekly/monthly reports

Mission(s) Served DoD Owner System	Link to AFHSC	Coverage/Completeness of Populations	Coverage/Completeness of Events Monitored	Quality/Accuracy	Timeliness (Frequency)
Biological weapons defense **USD(AT&L)/NCB, DTRA/JPEO** Joint Biological Agent Identification & Diagnostic System (**JBAIDS**)	GEIS (has funded flu assays)	350 worldwide locations (includes Navy/Army OCONUS Labs, Navy/Army/AF Preventive Medicine Units, Army Deployable Veterinary Units, Army Veterinary Food Service Teams, Navy ships)	• 16 pathogen surveillance assay kits are deployed covering 14 biological warfare agents. • 7 FDA cleared in vitro diagnostic kits- anthrax, tularemia, plague, q-fever, H5 avian flu, Influenza testing kits: flu A & B typing, flu A subtyping	Identification and diagnostic confirmation of biological agents	*Sample collection*: by partner lab *Data feeds*: not regular *Data analysis*: upon receipt
Force health protection, Biological weapons defense **Navy** Naval Medical Research Center lab (**NMRC**)	GEIS	NMRC is the central node for all Navy Research Labs, including OCONUS labs; specimens are received from labs	Specimen repository, including a variety of agents: • Respiratory (flu, adenoviruses, etc.) • Gastrointestinal (bacterial, viral) • Febrile and vector-borne pathogens	Hand-held assays, molecular diagnostics, confirmatory analysis	*Data collection*: supporting organization to provide validating resources to partner labs *Data feeds*: As required *Data analysis*: Reports are developed based on world events; publication/distribution frequency varies (e.g., quarterly, annually)

112

Mission(s) Served DoD Owner System	Link to AFHSC	Coverage/Completeness of Populations	Coverage/Completeness of Events Monitored	Quality/Accuracy	Timeliness (Frequency)
Force health protection, Global health security, Biological weapons defense **USD(AT&L)/DTRA/ JPEO/CBMS** Next Generation Diagnostic System (**NGDS**)	GEIS	Represents an effort to standardize new diagnostic platforms in all DoD CONUS and OCONUS support labs (~22 laboratories)	Similar to the JBAIDS in use; emerging pathogens, consumables (NCoV, H7N9)	Lab-confirmed	Vision of supporting laboratory characterization and pathogen discovery for surveillance and clinical diagnostics
Force health protection, Biological weapons defense **Army/MRMC** **USAMRIID**	GEIS / Partner Labs	Lab -- samples come from Chemical Biological Medical Systems (CBMS) within DTRA/JPEO	Anthrax, botulism, plague, Ebola and Marburg hemorrhagic fevers, hantavirus, ricin toxin, Staphylococcal enterotoxin B	National reference laboratory	_Sample collection:_ CBMS/DTRA/partner labs _Data feeds:_ as reported _Data analysis:_ quarterly and annually based surveillance reports
Global health security **Army/WRAIR** Viral Disease Branch-Genomic Center	GEIS	Receives influenza isolates from any DoD MHS or partner laboratory; isolate from patients with Severe Acute Respiratory infections or pneumonia	Deep-sequencing of influenza and other viruses - viral and influenza genomic shifts and drifts	Genetic sequencing	_Specimen collection:_ From DoD MHS or Partner Lab, Seasonally _Data feeds:_ Sent to NHRC, USAFSAM and GEIS for Vaccines and Related Biological Products Advisory Committee (FDA) _Data analysis:_ Reports received weekly, quarterly and annually based on surveillance type, project

113

Appendix D. GEIS Network and Partners

Table D.1. GEIS Network Countries, by Combatant Command and GEIS Syndromic Pillars Covered

Combatant Command	Country	Capacity Building	Antimicrob Resistance	Enteric illness	Febrile, Vector-borne	Malaria	Respiratory illness	Sexually-transmitted infections
USAFRICOM (n = 22)	Burkina Faso						X	
	Cameroon	X					X	X
	Cote d'Ivoire						X	
	Djibouti			X	X	X	X	X
	Gabon	X		X		X		
	Ghana			X	X	X	X*	X
	Kenya	X		X	X	X	X*	X
	Liberia			X	X	X		
	Libya						X	
	Mali						X*	
	Mauritania						X	
	Nigeria					X	X*	
	Seychelles	X						
	Sierra Leone				X			
	South Sudan			X	X			
	Sudan						X*	
	Tanzania				X			
	Togo			X			X	
	Uganda	X				X	X	
	Senegal						X*	
	South Africa						X*	
	Zimbabwe						X*	
USCENTCOM (n = 10)	Afghanistan						X*	
	Egypt	X		X	X	X	X*	
	Iraq						X*	
	Jordan		X				X*	
	Oman						X	
	Qatar						X	
	Yemen						X	
	Kuwait						X*	
	Pakistan						X*	
	Saudi Arabia						X*	
USEUCOM (n = 9)	Georgia				X		X	X
	Germany						X*	
	Russia						X*	
	Italy						X*	
	Kazakhstan						X*	
	Poland						X*	
	Serbia						X*	
	Turkey						X*	
	UK						X*	
USNORTHCOM	US	X	X	X	X		X	X

Combatant Command	Country	Capacity Building	Antimicrob Resistance	Enteric illness	Febrile, Vector-borne	Malaria	Respiratory illness	Sexually-transmitted infections
USPACOM (n = 22)	Australia					X	X*	
	Bhutan			X			X	
	Cambodia	X		X	X	X	X*	
	Japan				X			
	Korea				X		X*	
	Laos				X		X*	
	Mongolia				X		X	
	Nepal	X					X*	
	Philippines	X		X	X		X*	
	Soloman Islands					X		
	Thailand	X		X	X	X	X*	X
	Vanuatu					X		
	Vietnam					X	X*	
	Bangladesh						X*	
	Burma						X*	
	China						X*	
	India						X*	
	Indonesia						X*	
	Malaysia						X*	
	Singapore						X*	
	Sri Lanka						X*	
	Taiwan						X*	
USSOUTHCOM (n = 12)	Colombia				X		X*	
	Ecuador	X			X			
	Guatemala						X	
	Haiti					X		
	Honduras				X			
	Nicaragua						X	
	Paraguay				X			
	Peru	X	X	X	X	X	X*	X
	Chile						X*	
	El Salvador						X*	
	Mexico						X*	
	Venezuela						X*	

* Indicates countries where U.S. embassies receive test kits; see also Table C.1 in Appendix C, under Embassy-Based Respiratory Surveillance

Table D.2. Funded Labs in GEIS Network (Fiscal Year 2013)

Service or Type	Name (and Location)
Army	65th Medical Brigade (Korea)
	AFHSC (GEIS HQ, Maryland)
	AFRIMS (Thailand)
	Landstuhl Regional Medical Center (Germany)
	PHC Main (Maryland)
	PHCR-EUR (Germany)
	PHCR-SOUTH (Texas)
	San Antonio Military Medical Center (SAMMC, Texas)
	USAMRIID (HQ, Maryland)
	USAMRU-K (Kenya)
	USAMRU-G (Georgia)
	WRAIR - BAQC&RICK (includes Rickettsia, Maryland)
	WRAIR-ENTO (Entomology, Maryland)
	WRAIR ET (AAMI) (Australian Army Malaria Institute, Australia)
	WRAIR PM (Preventive Medicine, Maryland)
	WRAIR VD (Viral Diseases Branch, Maryland)
Navy	NAMRU-2 (Singapore)
	NAMRU-3 (Egypt)
	NAMRU-6 (Peru)
	Navy Environmental and Preventive Medicine Unit-2 (Virginia)
	NHRC (California)
	NMRC (Maryland)
	NMPDC (Navy Medicine Professional Development Center, Maryland)
Air Force	U.S. Air Force School of Aerospace Medicine (USAFSAM)
Other	Centers for Disease Control and Prevention (CDC)
	Global Viral Forecasting (now Metabiota)
	Imperial College London
	Johns Hopkins University Applied Physics Laboratory (JHUAPL)
	LOVELACE (National Laboratory, New Mexico)
	NASA
	Population Services International (PSI)
	SUNY Upstate
	University of Florida
	Uniformed Services University of the Health Sciences (DoD/USUHS, Maryland)

Appendix E. DMSS Data Feeds

Table E.1. DMSS Data Feeds

System	System Name	Type of Data	Frequency	Organization To/From	Org Acronym
ADMF	Active Duty Master File	Personnel Data	Monthly	Defense Manpower Data Center	DMDC
AFMES	Armed Forces Medical Examiner System	Casualty	Monthly	Armed Forces Medical Examiner System	AFMES
AFRESS	Air Force Reportable Events Surveillance System	Reportable Events	Weekly	U.S. Air Force School of Aerospace Medicine	USAFSAM
ASIMS	Aeromedical Services Info. Management Systems	Deployment Assessments	Weekly	Air Force Medical Support Agency	AFMSA
CDD_Army	Center for Disease Detection (Army)	HIV/Serologic data	Weekly	Center for Disease Detection (Army)	CDD
CDD_MEPS	Center for Disease Detection (MEPS)	HIV/Serologic data	Weekly	Center for Disease Detection (MEPS)	CDD
CDD_Navy	Center for Disease Detection (Navy)	HIV/Serologic data	Weekly	Center for Disease Detection (Navy)	CDD
CTS	Contingency Tracking System	Deployment Data	Monthly	Defense Manpower Data Center	DMDC
CTS_CIV	Contingency Tracking System (Civilians)	Deployment Data	Monthly	Defense Manpower Data Center	DMDC
DEERS	Defense Enrollment Eligibility Reporting Systems	Immunizations	Daily	Defense Manpower Data Center	DMDC
DHSS	Defense Health Services Systems	CAPER (Outpatient)	Daily	Tricare Management Activity	TMA
DHSS	Defense Health Services Systems	HL-7 Lab Chem	Daily	Tricare Management Activity	TMA
DHSS	Defense Health Services Systems	HL-7 Lab Micro	Daily	Tricare Management Activity	TMA
DHSS	Defense Health Services Systems	HL-7 Lab Path	Daily	Tricare Management Activity	TMA
DHSS	Defense Health Services Systems	HL-7 Pharm	Daily	Tricare Management Activity	TMA
DHSS	Defense Health Services Systems	Master Patient Index	Monthly	Tricare Management Activity	TMA
DHSS	Defense Health Services Systems	SIDR (Inpatient)	Monthly	Tricare Management Activity	TMA
DHSS	Defense Health Services Systems	TED_NI	Monthly	Tricare Management Activity	TMA
DHSS	Defense Health Services Systems	TED-I	Monthly	Tricare Management Activity	TMA
DRSi	Disease Reporting System (Army)	Reportable Events	Weekly	U.S. Army Public Health Command	USAPHC
eDHA	Electronic Deployment Health Assessment	Deployment Assessments	Daily	Navy and Marine Corps Public Health Center	NMCPHC
EPI_LAB	Epidemiology Laboratory	HIV/Serologic data	Weekly	U.S. Air Force School of Aerospace Medicine	USAFSAM

119

System	System Name	Type of Data	Frequency	Organization To/From	Org Acronym
LIMS	Laboratory Information Management System	HIV/Serologic data	Weekly	Walter Reed Army Institute of Research	WRAIR
MEPS	Military Entrance Processing Station	MEPS	Monthly	Military Entrance Processing Command	MEPCOM
NDRS	Navy Disease Reporting System	Reportable Events	Weekly	Navy and Marine Corps Public Health Center	NMCPHC
RCMF	Reserve Component Master File	Personnel Data	Monthly	Defense Manpower Data Center	DMDC
RIDES	Remote Information Data Entry System	Deployment Assessments	Daily	Army Medical Protection System	MEDPROS

Appendix F. Biosurveillance Outputs

Table F.1. Recurrent Reports Produced by AFHSC in Fiscal Year 2012

Type	Frequency	Name	Recipient	Versions	#/year
Disease	Weekly	DoD Communicable Disease	42	1	52
		JTF Communicable Disease	27	1	52
		Influenza Surveillance (during influenza season October–May)	108+Web	1	32
		Influenza-like Illness (ILI) Surveillance report (October–May)	1	1	32
		VA Influenza Surveillance Report* (October–May)	1	1	32
	Monthly	Malaria YTD Korea	1	1	12
		Monthly Malaria Case Finding Report	5	1	12
		Meningococcal Report Line Listing	1	1	12
	Annual	AFPMB Report for Arthropod Borne Hemorrhagic Fever	Web	1	1
		AFPMB Report for Mosquito Borne Encephalitis	Web	1	1
		AFPMB Report for Dengue/Hemorrhagic Fever	Web	1	1
		AFPMB Report for Lyme Disease	Web	1	1
		AFPMB Report for West Nile Fever	Web	1	1
		AFPMB Report for Leishmaniasis	Web	1	1
		Annual HIV Update	Web	1	1
Subtotal				15	243
Vaccine	Monthly	Smallpox and Anthrax Vaccine Adverse Events–Cardiac	1	1	12
		Reportable Events Vaccine Adverse Events (VAERS)	1	1	12
		Adenovirus Vaccine Monthly Safety Report	1	1	12
	Quarterly	Adenovirus Vaccine Quarterly Safety Report	1	1	4
Subtotal				4	40

Type	Frequency	Name	Recipient	Versions	#/year
Deployment	Monthly	Pre-Deployment Health Assessment (DD2795) Summary Report	50	2	24
		Post-Deployment Health Assessment (DD2796) Summary Report	50	2	24
		Post-Deployment Health Reassessment (DD2900) Summary Report	50	2	24
		Deployment Numbers Report	1	1	12
	Quarterly	Civilian Pre-Deployment Health Assessment (DD2795) Summary Report	1	1	4
		Civilian Post-Deployment Health Assessment Summary Report	2	1	4
		DoD Eye Injury	1	1	4
		DoD Hearing Injury Report	1	1	4
		Civilian Post-Deployment Health Reassessment Summary Report	1	1	4
		Deployment Health Compliance Report	2	4	16
		Deployment Health Civilian Compliance Report	50	1	4
		Deployment Health Report	2	1	4
	Semi-Annual	Army DD2900 Delinquency Report	3	1	2
	Annual	DoD Annual Eye Injury	1	1	1
		DoD Annual Hearing Injury	1	1	1
		USCG PHA, PDHA, PDHR	1	3	3
Subtotal				24	135
Mental Health	Monthly	DCoE TBI Diagnoses for DTM	1	1	12
		TBI Positive Screenings Line Listing	1	1	12
		USASOC Mental Health and TBI Monthly Report	1	1	12
		MHS Dashboard Measures Report (by condition)	1	1	12
		MHS Dashboard Measures (Service Specific)	1	1	12
		HA Mental Health Report	5	1	12
	Quarterly	USASOC Mental Health and TBI Quarterly Report	1	1	12
		HA TBI Report	5	2	8
		Defense and Veterans Brain Injury Center TBI Positive Screen Report	1	1	4
		DoD Consolidated TBI Healthcare Encounter Report	1	4	16
		AFSOC Mental Health and TBI Quarterly Report	1	1	12
		AFSOC Mental Health and TBI Annual Report	1	1	12
	Annual	Injury Installation Reports	Web	1	12
Subtotal				17	148

122

Type	Frequency	Name	Recipient	Versions	#/year
Injury	Monthly	Lost Duty Application	Web	1	12
		Force Health Protection Council Metrics	1	1	12
		Reserve Lost Duty Metrics	4	2	24
		Ill, Injured, and Wounded Report	1	1	12
		TRADOC Injury Report	7	2	24
		TMDS D&I Report	1	1	4
	Quarterly	USASOC Special Reportable Events	1	1	3
	Semi-Annual	Army Annual Injury Report	1	1	1
	Annual	USCG Burden of Disease	1	1	1
		TRADOC Heat Injury Report	1	1	1
		TRADOC Cold Injury Report	1	1	1
Subtotal				14	95
Special	Weekly	Weekly MedEvacs Report for DMDC	7	1	52
		Theater Medical Data Store (TMDS) Data Update Report	1	1	52
		USTRANSCOM Regulating and Command and Control Evacuation System (TRAC2ES) Data update - movement of sick or injured Members	1	1	52
	Monthly	DMSS Counts	1	1	12
		MHS Dashboard Measures	5	6	72
		Special Surveillance: Amputations, DVT, Leish, ARDs, TBI	1	1	12
		MSMR Special Surveillance Motor Vehicle Accidents	1	1	12
		MSMR Deployment Health Assessment	1	1	12
		Automated Neuropsychological Assessment Metrics (ANAM) Report	1	1	12
		MSMR Sentinel Reportable Events	1	1	12
		USEUCOM RMES Monthly Report	1	1	12
	Quarterly	Disease and Injury Distribution by Service	4	2	8
	Semi-Annual	DMISID Table (quality assurance report with location ID information)	1	1	2
	Annual	USCG RepEvent Report Table	1	1	1
		HA PTSD Monthly	5	2	24
Subtotal				22	347
Total				96	1,008

References

42 U.S.C. 5121 et seq. Chapter 68, *Disaster Relief.*

AFHSC—*See* Armed Forces Health Surveillance Center.

Armed Forces Health Surveillance Center, "Armed Forces Health Surveillance Center Concept of Operations (CONOPS) (DRAFT)," January 23, 2009.

———, "Stategic Plan for Fiscal Years 2013–2015," April 2013a.

———, "AFHSC Base Funding TMA MEDCOM," July 15, 2013b.

Camm, F., and B. M. Stecher, *Analyzing the Operation of Performance-Based Accountability Systems for Public Services*, Santa Monica, CA: RAND Corporation, TR-853, 2010. As of July 29, 2013:
http://www.rand.org/pubs/technical_reports/TR853.html

CDC—*See* Centers for Disease Control and Prevention.

Centers for Disease Control and Prevention, "Updated Guidelines for Evaluating Public Health Surveillance Systems: Recommendations from the Guidelines Working Group," *Morbitity and Mortality Weekly Report,* Vol. 50, No. RR-13, 2001.

———, "National Biosurveillance Strategy for Human Health, Version 2.0," February 2010. As of July 29, 2013:
http://www.cdc.gov/osels/pdf/NBSHH_v2.pdf

———, "Public Health Preparedness Capabilities: National Standards for State and Local Planning," March 2011. As of June 19, 2013:
http://www.cdc.gov/phpr/capabilities/

Defense Threat Reduction Agency, "Cooperative Threat Reduction Program Fiscal Year (FY) 2014 Budget Estimates," 2013. As of June 19 2013:
http://comptroller.defense.gov/defbudget/fy2014/budget_justification/pdfs/01_Operation_an d_Maintenance/O_M_VOL_1_PART_2/CTR_OP-5.pdf

Department of Defense, "Department of Defense Agency Financial Report for FY 2012," 2012a. As of June 13, 2013:
http://comptroller.defense.gov/afr/fy2012/3-Financial_Section.pdf

———, *Agency Financial Report for FY2012*, November 2012. As of 13 June 2013:
http://comptroller.defense.gov/afr/fy2012/3-Financial_Section.pdf

———, "Fiscal Year (FY) 2014 Budget RDT&E Programs (R-1) - Unclassified," April 2013a, pp. D-18. As of July 29, 2013:
http://comptroller.defense.gov/defbudget/fy2014/fy2014_r1.pdf

———, "Fiscal Year (FY) 2014 President's Budget Submission, Chemical Biological Defense Program, Justification Book Volume 4 of 4: Research, Development, Test & Evaluation, Defense-Wide," April 2013b. As of 17 June 2013:
http://comptroller.defense.gov/

————, "Fiscal Year (FY) 2014 President's Budget Submission, Defense Health Program," April 2013c. As of 17 June 2013:
http://comptroller.defense.gov/

Department of Defense Directive 3025.18, "Defense Support of Civil Authorities," December 29, 2010.

Department of Defense Directive 6200.04, "Force Health Protection (FHP)," April 2007.

Department of Defense Directive 6490.02E, "Comprehensive Health Surveillance," February 8, 2012, February 8, 2012.

DHA Public Health sub Work Group, "Public Health sub Work Group briefing part 3- future state structures," May 16, 2013.

DoD—*See* Department of Defense.

DoDD—*See* Department of Defense Directive.

DTRA—*See* Defense Threat Reduction Agency.

Greenfield, V., V. Williams, and E. Eiseman, *Using Logic Models for Strategic Planning and Evaluation: Application to the National Center for Injury Prevention and Control*, Santa Monica, Calif.: The RAND Corporation, TR-370-NCIPC, 2006. As of July 29, 2013:
http://www.rand.org/pubs/technical_reports/TR370.html

HHS—*See* United States Department of Health and Human Services.

Homeland Security Presidential Directive 21, "Public Health and Medical Preparedness," October 18, 2007. As of July 29, 2013:
http://www.hsdl.org/?collection/stratpol&id=pd&pid=gwb

HSPD 21—*See* Homeland Security Presidential Directive 21.

Ijaz, K., E. Kasowski, R. R. Arthur, F. J. Angulo, and S. F. Dowell, "International Health Regulations--what gets measured gets done," *Emerging Infectious Diseases,* Vol. 18, No. 7, July 2012, pp. 1054–1057. As of July 29, 2013:
http://www.ncbi.nlm.nih.gov/pubmed/22709593

Institute of Medicine, *The Future of the Public's Health in the 21st Century*, Washington, DC: National Academies Press, 2002.

Joint Publication 1-02, "Department of Defense Dictionary of Military and Associated Terms," April 2013.

Joint Staff/J-8, "Joint DOTmLPF-P Change Recommendation for Biosurveillance, Version 1.9.3 (DRAFT)," March 27, 2013.

McNabb, S. J. N., S. Chungong, M. Ryan, T. Wuhib, P. Nsubuga, W. Alemu, V. Carande-Kulis, and G. Rodier, "Conceptual Framework of Public Health Surveillance and Action and Its Application in Health Sector Reform," *BMC Public Health,* Vol. 2, No. 2, 2002.

Moore, M., "The Global Dimensions of Public Health Preparedness and Implications for US Action," *American Journal of Public Health,* Vol. 102, No. 6, June 2012, pp. e1–7. A of July 29, 2013:
http://www.ncbi.nlm.nih.gov/pubmed/22515870

Moore, M., E. Chan, N. Lurie, A. G. Schaefer, D. M. Varda, and J. A. Zambrano, "Strategies to Improve Global Influenza Surveillance: A Decision Tool for Policymakers," *BMC Public Health,* Vol. 8, 2008, p. 186. As of July 29, 2013:
http://www.ncbi.nlm.nih.gov/pubmed/18507852

Moore M., D. J. Dausey, B. Phommasack, S. Touch, G. Lu, S. Lwin Nyein, K. Ungchusak, N. D. Vung, and M. K. Oo, "Sustainability of Sub-Regional Disease Surveillance Networks," *Global Health Governance,* Vol. V, No. 2, Spring 2012.

Moore, Melinda, Elisa Eisemann, Gail Fischer, Stuart S. Olmsted, Preethi R. Sama, and John A. Zambrano, *Harnessing Full Value from the DoD Serum Repository and the Defense Medical Surveillance System,* Santa Monica, Calif.: The RAND Corporation, MG-875-A, 2010. As of July 29, 2013:
http://www.rand.org/pubs/monographs/MG875.html

Nsubuga, P., M. E. White, S. B. Thacker, M. A. Anderson, S. B. Blount, C. V. Broome, T. Chiller, V. Espitia, R. Imtiaz, D. Sosin, D. F. Stroup, and R. V. Tauxe, "Chapter 53 - Public Health Surveillance: A Tool for Targeting and Monitoring Interventions," in D. T. Jamison, J. G. Breman, A. R. Measham et al., eds., *Disease Control Priorities in Developing Countries,* Washington, DC: World Bank, 2006.

Office of the Secretary of Defense, "Memorandum: Interim Guidance for Implementing the National Strategy for Biosurveillance," June 13, 2013.

OSD—*See* Office of the Secretary of Defense.

PDD—*See* Presidential Decision Directive.

Presidential Decision Directive NSTC-7, "Emerging Infectious Diseases," June 12, 1996.

Presidential Decision Directive 2, "National Strategy for Countering Biological Threats," November 2009.

Schick, A., "Planning-Programming-Budgeting System: A Symposium. The Road to PPB: The Stages of Budget Reform," *Public Administration Review,* December 1996, p. 244.

Shelton, S. R., C. D. Nelson, A. W. McLees, K. Mumford, and C. Thomas, "Building Performance-Based Accountability With Limited Empirical Evidence: Performance Measurement for Public Health Preparedness," *Disaster Medicine and Public Health Preparedness,* Vol. 00, No. 00, 2013.

Thacker, S. B., "Historical Development," in S. T. Teutsch and R. E. Churchill, eds., *Principles and Practice of Public Health Surveillance,* New York: Oxford University Press, 2000.

United States Department of Health and Human Services, Office of Disease Prevention and Health Promotion, *Healthy People 2020,* Washington, DC. As of June 19, 2013:
http://www.healthypeople.gov/2020/topicsobjectives2020/

United States Department of Health and Human Services, "National Health Security Strategy of the United States of America," December 2009. As of June 17, 2013:
http://www.phe.gov/Preparedness/planning/authority/nhss/strategy/Documents/nhss-final.pdf

White House, "National Security Strategy," March 2006. As of July 29, 2013:
http://georgewbush-whitehouse.archives.gov/nsc/nss/2006/index.html

———, "National Security Strategy," May 2010. As of July 29, 2013:
http://www.whitehouse.gov/sites/default/files/rss_viewer/national_security_strategy.pdf

———, "National Strategy for Biosurveillance," July 2012. As of April 22, 2013:
http://www.whitehouse.gov/sites/default/files/National_Strategy_for_Biosurveillance_July_2012.pdf

———, "Memorandum: Fiscal Year 2015 Budget Guidance for Countering Biological Threats Resource Priorities," June 27, 2013.

White House National Security Staff, Emerging Pandemic Threats Sub-Interagency Policy Committee, "Promoting Global Health Security: Guidance and Principles for U.S. Government Departments and Agencies to Strengthen IHR Core Capacities Internationally," June, 2011.

WHO—*See* World Health Organization.

World Health Organization, *International Health Regulations (2005), 2nd ed*, Geneva, 2008. As of July 29, 2013:
http://whqlibdoc.who.int/publications/2008/9789241580410_eng.pdf